Praise for

Find Your Stride

"*Find Your Stride* is the book that the exercise and fitness world needs right now. Emily Rudow sorts through the mess of hype and false promises to provide a clear, actionable, and researched-backed guide that will help you live a healthier, happier life."

—Steve Magness, author of *Peak Performance*

"Emily Rudow is the perfect person to tackle sustainable nutrition and training. In a world full of 'hacks,' silver bullets, and quick fixes—none of which work, of course—this book provides an honest and refreshing look at how to actually be your best, as well as concrete and evidence-based steps to take you there."

—Brad Stulberg, author of *The Practice of Groundedness*

"In *Find Your Stride*, Emily Rudow does a fantastic job blending common sense and the most up-to-date research to provide fitness guidance that refreshingly doesn't include gimmicks or quick fixes but does include long-term sustainability. The information is clear, and the advice is actionable and research-based but never bogs down the reader. If we had more books like this, the world would be a healthier, happier place."

—Eric Helms, PhD, CSCS, research fellow at the
Sports Performance Research Institute New Zealand,
Auckland University of Technology

FIND YOUR STRIDE

A Personalized Path to Sustainable
Nutrition and Training

EMILY RUDOW

RIVER GROVE
BOOKS

This book is intended as a reference volume only, not as a medical manual. The information given here is designed to help you make informed decisions about your health. It is not intended as a substitute for any treatment that may have been prescribed by your doctor. If you suspect that you have a medical problem, you should seek competent medical help. You should not begin a new health regimen without first consulting a medical professional.

Published by River Grove Books
Austin, TX
www.rivergrovebooks.com

Distributed by River Grove Books

Design and composition by Greenleaf Book Group and Mimi Bark
Cover design by Greenleaf Book Group and Mimi Bark
Cover images used under license from ©Shutterstock.com/Kzlmax;
©Shutterstock.com/Sucha Kittiwararat; ©Shutterstock.com/AlexandrBognat

Publisher's Cataloging-in-Publication data is available.

Print ISBN: 978-1-63299-519-3

eBook ISBN: 978-1-63299-520-9

First Edition

To my fam

Contents

Introduction

Just one semester into starting my undergraduate degree at Wilfrid Laurier University, I was already on the verge of dropping out. During that fall of 2007, my grades in my core courses barely made the cut, and I was awarded my worst grade ever (a D– in microeconomics). On top of my miserable grades, I was grappling with body-image issues. From the time I graduated high school to the end of my first year of college, I had gained an extra 10 pounds—not quite the "freshman 15," but close. The self-consciousness I felt about my body was debilitating. Comparing myself to others was a regular occurrence, I drank and partied in excess, and I suffered from extreme bouts of anxiety. In short, my first year was hell, but somehow, I made it through.

That summer I worked at a frozen yogurt shop and ate my way through my misery with frequent snack breaks of chocolate/vanilla swirl topped with Skor and Oreo. Those were a delicious and terrible few months as I sunk deeper into myself.

In high school, I had struggled with confidence issues surrounding my weight and appearance. I cared so much about what other people thought. It wasn't until the end of the summer before my second year of college that I realized this wasn't the life I wanted for myself—I decided that I'd had enough. My body shaming had reached its limits, and I wanted to take control. I no longer wanted to use food as a crutch and inadvertently as fuel for my own internal body shaming. I was ready and willing to do whatever it took to lose weight and *finally* feel comfortable in my own skin.

I wish I could share with you that the start of my fitness journey was driven by a majestic moment—an epiphany on a longer run or a tragic loss that propelled me into a life-changing plan to deal with my deep, emotional pain. Sorry to disappoint, but my beginning is anticlimactic; the inception for me was when I walked into a health and supplement store. I bought a big tub of protein powder and grabbed some fish oils—two supplements I thought would aid me on my new fitness journey. On my way out, a little pamphlet caught my eye. I picked it up and saw that it contained a 22-minute treadmill workout. This little piece of paper, my friends, was the starting point.

Because I'm an extreme kind of gal, I went all in on a new fitness and nutrition plan that I created for myself. I gobbled up every resource I could find, starting with a very outdated book called *Fit for Life* (written in 1985). I developed strict rules that I had to adhere to. I would allow myself to have only what Brian Tracy, the prolific self-development guru, would deem "safe" foods—those that didn't include excessive amounts of the "three white poisons": salt, refined sugar, and white flour. I could consume only foods marked "fat free." And alcohol? Well, that was completely off the table. I would allow myself one to two servings of carbohydrates (in the forms of bread, rice, pasta, wraps, etc.) per day. I could eat as many fruits and vegetables as I wanted, as outlined in *Fit for Life*. Basically, I took a mishmash of random suggestions I heard or read on the internet and decided that this is what I would follow. I didn't track any sort of calories or macros back then.

My fitness plan was equally strict. I committed to going to the gym five days per week and would do 20 minutes of cardio three times per week and resistance training broken out as follows: arms and back two times per week, and legs and core two times per week. I researched exercises on the internet and started working out at my university's gym. I followed this plan religiously for months. *And guess what?* It worked. I started to lose weight, and after a few months, I saw dramatic changes in my body. My friends started to notice too. I received compliments and accolades for my efforts, and as a side effect, my confidence skyrocketed. I started doing better in school. Well, not my finance and accounting courses—I still sucked at math.

All was good in the world, except one tiny little thing: I had formed this rigidity that allowed for no flexibility with my eating or fitness. I also developed a visceral fear: I was terrified that if I had one little slip-up, ate one "bad" thing, all the weight would return. I'm not even kidding you. I am educated and would define myself as a moderately intelligent person, but this was my train of thought. The obsessiveness with my diet and rigidity in my workouts inevitably led to an eating disorder. I started eliminating or drastically reducing my carb intake and replaced those carbs with carrots. Seriously, carrots. I ate so many damn carrots that the beta-carotene started turning my skin orange. I was trapped in my own self-made prison, and finding a healthy balance was an ongoing struggle.

It took me a long time to break free of this trap and allow myself to become more flexible with both my diet and my exercise. While body transformation (building muscle and losing fat) was my goal at the start, I started discovering deeper meaning in my training. Running was a way for me to relieve stress, reduce my anxiety, clear my head, and work through difficult problems; that time I carved out for myself on a regular basis was my own little sanctuary.

I ran in the morning and experienced the quotidian runner's high, sustaining the euphoric feeling and high energy for the entirety of the day. I slowly started getting better at my 22-minute treadmill workout, upping my levels and doing the same amount of mileage faster and faster. Running was a mechanism I could use to challenge myself, and most importantly, it made me *feel* good. I also enjoyed resistance training and the meditative state I'd experience in focusing on a single rep at a time. I got stronger and started to see palpable changes in my physique; my body took on a more toned appearance.

As my fitness knowledge increased, I allowed for a bit more flexibility with my diet—now knowing that a single slice of pizza wouldn't make me balloon. I slowly allowed more of my former forbidden foods back into my life, which didn't come served with a side of guilt and shame. I even got my personal training certificate in my third year of college.

I carried this new lifestyle with me after I graduated and was able to sustain my fitness regimen. I ran my first half marathon (13.1 miles) in 2010 and my first marathon (26.2 miles) in 2012. From there, I kept running as an integral part of my life because I loved it. From a physique perspective, however, I hit a plateau. I stopped reading and experimenting on myself, got lazy, and continued to follow the same old plan that had worked in the past. I was performing the same exercises day in and day out, so I was able to maintain my weight, for the most part. But my results became stagnant, and my physique stayed relatively the same.

That is, until 2016, when I unintentionally began a path of self-experimentation that ultimately transformed my life. It was another rough year for me. I had just gotten out of a four-year relationship and quit my full-time job at an advertising agency to pursue a venture in the random world of manufacturing protective base-layer apparel for hockey players. My ex also happened to be my business partner, which added another layer of complication. The heartache, combined with the struggles of trying to make a living within the first year of a start-up, caused me to have my first series of panic attacks. For several months of this tumultuous year, I struggled to pay my rent and could barely even afford groceries. Self-employment wasn't all it was cracked up to be. At the end of the year, the panic attacks led to a full mental breakdown, in which I felt so paralyzed that I could barely work.

With the support of my amazing family and friends, I was finally able to pick myself up and move forward. I prioritized my self-care by focusing on activities that nourished me, like reading and meditating. One of the books I happened to pick up in late 2016 sparked an idea that changed the trajectory of my life. *The Happiness of Pursuit*, by Chris Guillebeau, presents the concept of questing—how undertaking quests can add more meaning and purpose to our lives. Guillebeau describes a quest as a long-term goal or objective that's deeply personal to us and that sparks a sense of adventure and challenge in our lives. Guillebeau's own quest, and perhaps his motivation behind the book, was to travel to all 193 countries.

I was inspired, to say the least. While I didn't have any long-term quests in mind at the time, I did form my own mini version. I challenged myself to run 10 kilometers every day for the month of January. I made it through the month with 310 kilometers under my belt. In addition to the sense of accomplishment, there were other side effects worth noting: I gained confidence, knowing that I could stick to a commitment I set for myself, and I realized how quickly the body can adapt to increases in daily mileage (before the challenge I ran an average of only 5–6 kilometers most days). I developed more self-discipline, which translated into other areas of my life. Most importantly, I felt happier. I started to feel like myself again.

A few months went by, and I was itching for another challenge. Something bigger. Something better. Perhaps, even, a world-record-breaking attempt. While I was out for a run one day, I came up with an idea of doubling the distance while increasing the duration of the challenge. I made it official in May 2017: I would attempt to break a world record by running the half-marathon distance (21.1 kilometers/13.1 miles) every day for the most consecutive days. The women's world record was 61 days at the time (according to *Guinness World Records*), so I set a goal to run 70 days. I coined the name #RUN70 for the challenge, and to make it even more meaningful, I simultaneously set a goal to raise $10,000 for the Canadian Cancer Society. By taking the challenge one day at a time, building a supportive community that provided encouraging words, and experimenting with different recovery techniques, I broke the world record, hit my goal of 70 half marathons, and ran for a few extra days, rounding off the challenge on day 74.

I think day 74 was the day my real quest began. Since then, I have never taken a rest day and am still running an average of five miles every day as I write this over four years later. After the dopamine high from the challenge wore off, life returned to normal. I went back to my regular strength training regimen—repeating the same exercises day in and day out, not seeing any real palpable changes in my physique. I, once again, slipped back into a place of complacency and stagnation.

In 2019, another long-term relationship with someone I deeply cared about ended. To deal with the familiar and awful feelings accompanying a breakup, I wanted a big change. I actively started to pursue knowledge that would help me reach new fitness levels and could spark significant changes in my body composition. I started performing some formal self-experiments, documenting each change I made to my nutrition or training and recording how it affected my body, performance, mood, and energy levels. Over the course of only a few months, I started putting on some serious muscle definition, and my body fat began to dissipate. I saw more vascularity in my arms and legs. Over time, I slowly but surely let go of my old routine and embraced an entirely new one.

Now, I run regular self-experiments testing different calorie/macro intakes, nutrition timing strategies, and training splits—discovering *my own truths* through experimentation. I like to think of myself as an explorer—always open to evaluating new ideas that interest me and then incorporating what resonates with my lifestyle and tossing out the rest. Rinse and repeat. In this book, I want to teach you the same framework that can help you build lean muscle, lose body fat, and sustain a fitness routine and nutrition plan you actually enjoy over the long term—one that's uniquely tailored to you.

I've read hundreds of fitness and nutrition books, devoured countless scientific journals and PubMed articles, and watched innumerable hours of YouTube videos. The main takeaway I've drawn from my research is this: science in this industry is constantly evolving—sometimes at such a rapid pace, it's hard to keep up. Studies are constantly disproving other studies, so it's difficult to stay on top of the latest and, more important, most credible information. Adding another layer of complexity is that so many subjects are controversial. Credible fitness professionals are debating each other on topics like how much protein people really need or how intense our training sessions should be. Further, fitness is full of what blogger Nat Eliason calls "artificial complexity"—that is, taking the simple and purposely making it overly complex, usually with a motive (i.e., selling products and services that promise a simple solution to a supposedly complex problem).[1] We're duped into believing that the more complicated the plan, the more valuable and effective it will be.

My method is rooted in solid scientific research, personal anecdotes, and the mindset to discover my own truths. In this book, I draw not only from my own experience but also from credible fitness professionals and industry experts and the most up-to-date scientific literature. I also present multiple arguments on controversial issues—and sometimes I give my own recommendations—but always, and you'll notice this is a common thread throughout this book, I will point you toward conducting your own experiments.

WHAT YOU'LL GET OUT OF *FIND YOUR STRIDE*

I wrote *Find Your Stride* for people who have put effort into their training and nutrition for the most part but are frustrated because their efforts don't result in the transformative changes they really want—for people, like me, who crave the correct knowledge to get them where they want to go. This book is also for people who have struggled to stick with a nutrition or training plan long enough to see the desired results. Maybe you've tried many plans, stuck with them for a bit (as they started to work), but realized they weren't viable for the long term—either they were too boring, too restrictive (sparking feelings of deprivation), or the training was too intense (workouts felt like too much work too often).

Find Your Stride is about turning information into action. This book will help you build confidence from transforming your body and uncover the deeper, more intrinsic reasons for why you train, to build sustainable fitness for life.

People think they want to be told exactly what to do: the winning formula to achieve holistic well-being; the right recipe; the plan that will help them lose fat, build muscle, and increase energy levels. Most plans are rigid, with specific rules and principles to adhere to (eat this, don't eat that, do these exercises, don't do those), and don't have the flexibility to account for every individual's needs. When we veer off the path and don't fit the specific mold laid out by health gurus, we get discouraged and quit. But each and every one of us needs our own *unique* program—a program that's flexible and ever changing to suit our evolving lifestyle and preferences. Rapper 50 Cent and Robert Greene write in *The 50th Law*, "Understand: you are one of a kind. Your character traits are a kind of chemical mix that will never be repeated in history."[2]

Understanding that there is no such thing as a universal plan for everyone, I present in these pages an unconventional approach to fitness and a digestible amalgamation of the latest research in nutrition, exercise science, and psychology to give you the simple tools to transform your body and mind. The book offers pragmatic advice on how to craft individualized, sustainable training and nutrition plans to see real, palpable changes in your physique—more lean muscle mass and less body fat—and stick with said plans over the long haul.

Find Your Stride is not about following one plan to "arrive"; it's about being open to lifelong experimentation: learning, trying, tweaking, refining, and finding, through self-discovery, an individualized plan that's right for you. It's about doing small actions each day and conducting mini-experiments that compound into material changes over time.

In this book, I challenge you to look inward by providing the framework to find deeper meaning in your goals—a hallmark of building consistency. If you position yourself as an explorer, you can't fail and sabotage yourself. You're building a foundation to learn and grow, which is key to sustaining your fitness journey over the long term.

I encourage you to take the information that resonates with you and apply it to your routine. Being open minded and receptive to new information (even if it goes against your long-held beliefs) will be one of the most challenging tasks I ask of you. Equipped with the knowledge in this book, and your openness to trial and error, you can run your own experiments, track your progress, and gain the experience to propel you forward in your fitness journey.

Find Your Stride starts with the topic of mindset—letting go of old assumptions that are no longer serving you. I then dive into the topic of motivation and the latest theories on where long-term motivation comes from and how to use both intrinsic motivation for long-term sustainability and extrinsic rewards for short-term spurts of effort. Next, I cover how to develop important habits to set you up for a lifetime of success and self-experimentation. Then, we go over fitness goals—how to set them and what to watch out for.

The second and third parts of the book cover nutrition and training, respectively. In each part, I provide the building blocks and knowledge you need to hit your aesthetic physique goals. I dispel some myths and take some deep dives into a few of the more complex and controversial nutrition and fitness issues. You'll learn how to craft your own training and nutrition plans to achieve your individualized goals.

The final part is on sustainability—how to get back on the path when you fall off, how to deal with the bad days, the benefits of adopting a mindfulness practice, and some warnings and potential pitfalls when starting out any new fitness or nutrition plan.

I expect you to scrutinize this book—in fact, I encourage it. My goal is to provide you with a guide, rather than a gospel. I don't expect you to accept everything I write at face value, but rather, consider the information, apply it to your own life (through experimentation), and develop your own personal truths. The main point I want you to take away from this book is this: every plan we have must be catered uniquely to us.

While this book focuses on the fitness realm, the principles will translate well in all other aspects of your life. Feeling physically fit and healthy can provide you with the confidence to succeed financially, in your career, in relationships, and in other areas.

A FEW DISCLAIMERS

In all my published fitness articles, I always start off with a few disclaimers, and this book is no different. First, I am a white, able-bodied cisgender woman, and when I express my personal experience with a particular idea, I am speaking through this lens. I realize there are gender differences in how to optimally train, and when warranted, I call these out. In addition, there are racial differences and considerations when it comes to diet culture and fat loss; in my "Further Reading" section at the back of the book, I suggest specific BIPOC authors and educators who are much better equipped on this topic than I am. Second, for topics on which I don't have any direct experience to contribute as a cisgender white woman, I present unbiased information from credible sources and some of the latest studies. In sum, I don't believe fitness is binary; it's not black and white. There are a million shades of gray. I avoid telling you exactly what to do and encourage you to use what you want, toss out the rest, and check out the additional resources at the back of this book.

While writing this book was a rewarding experience, it was an overwhelming process at times, so keeping the main goal of helping others in mind throughout some of the more grueling days kept me going. I'm proud of how *Find Your Stride* came together and genuinely hope it helps you. I encourage you to get in touch; candid feedback (good or bad) is important to me. You can email me directly from the contact form on my website (https://emilyrudow.com/contact) or join my community on Instagram at https://www.instagram.com/emilyrudow.

So, without further ado, let's dive in.

PART I

————

MINDSET

CHAPTER 1

Changing Your Mindset

If knowledge is power, knowing what we don't know is wisdom.
—ADAM GRANT, *Think Again*

Right now, you may have beliefs, judgments, or a particular mindset toward fitness. Most likely, you've developed some strong opinions along your health and wellness journey. Some of these beliefs may have developed from firsthand experience, while others may have been ingrained in you by your social circle, articles or books you've read, videos you've watched, or the habits you formed during childhood. Each and every one of us has a unique lens that we see the world through, which is largely shaped by our environment.

Our beliefs can be great; they can guide us into action, act as a foundation for our value system, help us accomplish our goals, and push us to make meaningful changes in our life. But they also have the potential to keep us stuck in a state of complacency and stagnation. If you want your body to change, your mind needs to follow suit.

To change our mindset, we need to break free from the mindsets that are no longer serving us. Personal experience is one of the most difficult frames of reference to break free from. How many times have you tried a diet plan, seen tangible results, and then told everyone you know how effective that diet plan is? Since you saw the results, you now believe it's a universal truth. This happens to all of us, but how much value can we attribute to a focus group of one?

Restricting my carbs made me lose weight, but it took a toll on my mental health. I felt like garbage, and to be frank, I started treating others like garbage. Because I had experienced weight loss from sticking to a low-carb diet, I believed this was the only tried and trusted way to lose weight. This belief was ingrained in me for years.

This chapter reviews the more recent (and popularized) mindsets and how they may be holding you back from hitting your fitness goals. We'll then go over the importance of unlearning mindsets and how to take ego out of the equation. This is some important groundwork to cover before you progress through the remainder of this book.

GROWTH AND FIXED MINDSETS

The principles of *growth* and *fixed* mindsets were developed and popularized in psychologist Carol Dweck's book *Mindset: The New Psychology of Success*. She explains that a mindset is a self-perception or theory that someone holds about themselves.[1] She then looks at how our mindsets can have a profound impact on our personal relationships, academic and professional successes, how we acquire skills, and so on.

A fixed mindset is a binary way of perceiving yourself and, in Dweck's words, it is "believing that your qualities are carved in stone."[2] Believing that physically fit people are genetically gifted or that you're fat and nothing you do can change that is an example of thinking with a fixed mindset.[3] This mindset also assumes that success is a by-product of talent alone. The limitations of holding these fixed ideals about ourselves include shying away from challenges or not taking the necessary steps to learn and improve; predetermining every "risk" will result in failure before we even begin. Admiring the bodies of fitness models on Instagram or watching a stellar athlete like Michael Phelps on television, we assume their physiques or abilities are innate traits.

In contrast, a growth mindset operates on the inverse. People with this mindset believe they can develop their skills through sheer hard work, and they have an ardent love for learning, despite where they start from or innate talents they may or may not possess. Dweck writes, "This *growth mindset* is based on the belief that your basic qualities are things you can cultivate through your efforts, your strategies, and help from others. Although people may differ in every which way—in their initial talents, aptitudes, interests of temperaments—everyone can change and grow through application and experience."[4]

Harnessing our strengths through hard work, learning, and perseverance will ultimately help propel us forward. A growth mindset can be learned and is fundamental in achieving any type of fitness goal. While it is true that some people might have a bit more of a head start because of genetics or their social location, we can all achieve our fitness goals by classifying ourselves as individuals in flux: we are evolving creatures who are open to learning and change as we progress throughout our lives.

Why is this important? Wherever your starting point is, remember that it isn't fixed. You will make progress and can actively work toward any fitness or health goals you set out for yourself; you just have to put in the work! But you know that already. And as an additional note, if you haven't done a fitness or training program before—or it has been awhile—it's always good practice to speak with your health care provider before getting started.

UNLEARNING AND RELEARNING

I've held a consistent fitness routine for 14 years now, and over the course of this journey, I've experienced both dramatic body transformations and long periods of stagnation. I noticed a little definition but no material changes for years. It wasn't until I went through the process of unlearning—practicing humility, stepping away from my long-held beliefs about fitness, and adopting a new routine—that I was able to make significant gains in muscle definition and vascularity while decreasing my body fat.

I used to believe that I would lose muscle if I didn't perform the same exercises in a particular order the same days each week. I used to think that eating very few carbs and close to zero fats would be the only way for me to lose weight. I also used to believe, after watching *Willy Wonka and the Chocolate Factory* (when I was six years old, to be clear), that I would turn into a blueberry if I chewed gum; luckily, my parents convinced me otherwise!

As silly as it may sound, I was scared that I would lose all the progress I made with my training if I tweaked the smallest thing—that changing even a single variable in my routine could throw me into a tailspin. This hypothesis, however, turned out to be unfounded, and by overhauling my routine entirely, I was finally able to improve my running performance and alter my body composition to a level I had never experienced before.

I also considered my diet relatively healthy. I would at the time guesstimate that around 80% of the food I ate could be classified as "nutritionally dense," but I still struggled to lose body fat. I didn't get it—I thought I was doing everything right. Avocado toast was supposed to catapult me into holistic health and well-being. By starting to track my portions and what I was putting into my body, I realized that I was in a caloric surplus most days (eating more calories than I expended). I forced myself out of a place of complacency by seeking out new information, validating that information through experimentation, and making any necessary tweaks along the way. The point I'm trying to make is that we need to acknowledge that we don't know everything. Adam Grant writes, "In a turbulent world, there's another set of cognitive skills that might matter more [than intelligence]: the ability to rethink and unlearn."[5] Clearly, you're reading this book because you want to make a change, in whatever capacity that might be. You may have some sort of fitness goal (or multiple goals): gaining lean muscle and definition, losing body fat, or simply incorporating more movement into your life. What I ask while you continue to read this book is that you open your mind. As mentioned in the introduction, I don't want you to take everything I say as gospel. I'm anything but dogmatic—and you should be too when it comes to fitness. Rather, consider the information, think about what resonates with your own life and routine, and apply that. Experiment and tweak until you find a program that works for you.

EGO

You have to start somewhere. When I first started running, it was a struggle. Running for any length of time after the ten-minute mark was met with frequent stops, lots of walking breaks, and heavy breathing that could put your dad's snoring to shame. We all have a starting point when we dip our toes into uncharted waters and have to accept that we're not going to be experts automatically. Even those who were born with a precocious talent have to start somewhere. Whenever I attend a yoga class, I hide at the back of the class so no one can see how poor my flexibility is. Like most of us, my ego falls back on comfort—pursuing activities that I feel confident tackling, and shying away from anything new. Because "newness" comes with uncertainty. When I'm bad at something, my ego takes a beating.

Ego is one of the reasons we avoid embarking on new challenges, shy away from testing a new fitness class, or avoid signing up for a gym membership; the embarrassment of not knowing what you're doing can be paralyzing. To be fair, gyms can be full of judgment. They can be a meat market of grunts, slammed weights, people comparing themselves to others, and cheesy pickup lines. However, judgment doesn't live just in the gym; it's all around us, and it's important to ground yourself in knowing that this is *your* journey.

A passage from Steve Pavlina's book *Personal Development for Smart People* really stuck with me. Pavlina also discusses it on his blog, explaining that if we don't have the experience or credentials when approaching new situations, we should position ourselves as explorers.[6] We are always looking to grow and evolve, whether we're just starting out or we're 10 years deep into our journey. An explorer accepts that a starting point is evergreen; we can always learn and do more to improve.

I like this perspective and use it whenever I try a new activity. I reassure myself that it's okay to not master something right off the bat; I can always explore tactics and techniques to get better. Not to sound rudimentary, but practice really is the best improvement principle. I like to keep things light and fun. I make fun of myself a lot for screwing up. When I was doing a 30-day vegetarian challenge, you should have seen my first spirulina smoothie bowl attempt—how do influencers do it? My mom walked into the kitchen after I assembled my artful bowl and said, verbatim, "Holy shit, Emmy, that looks disgusting." We both laughed, and I decided to try to assemble an easier bowl on my next attempt.

In Ryan Holiday's book *Ego Is the Enemy*, he explains what happens when ego is removed from the equation:

> When we remove ego, we're left with what is real. What replaces ego is humility, yes—but rock-hard humility and confidence. Whereas ego is artificial, this type of confidence can hold weight. Ego is stolen. Confidence is earned. Ego is self-anointed, its swagger is artifice. One is girding yourself, the other gaslighting. It's the difference between potent and poisonous.[7]

At the end of the day, practice and ongoing work are the vehicles for personal growth. If we put our egos aside and stay open to learning from others, then we allow space for new ideas, perspectives, and challenges to emerge. So, whether you're already a seasoned gym-goer or just starting out, know that the material I present to you will probably require you to step out of the realm of the ego and adopt a new mentality when it comes to building out a fitness regimen. It's so easy to skim over information and say to yourself, "I know this already"—thanks, ego. I encourage you to step outside yourself and try some of the experiments or new methodologies in this book in your own routine. Don't just take my word for it; experience will help solidify what's true to you, which leads me to my next topic, the explorer mindset.

THE EXPLORER MINDSET

As previously mentioned, I like to think of my mindset as one of an explorer; that is, I take a more active role in my learning through self-experimentation, fueled by genuine curiosity. This is the mindset of a scientist: I'm devising a hypothesis, running self-experiments, and then tweaking, refining, and duplicating tests in the lab (a.k.a. the kitchen and gym) until I find the solution.

I define my existing nutrition and fitness regimen as a Frankenstein plan. I do research, test new theories, and apply bits and pieces to my routine. I don't follow one specific diet or one specific training plan. I mix different aspects and create something entirely new and uniquely *moi*.

This mindset applies not only to fitness but to other endeavors as well. If you start on a new self-made plan and position yourself as an explorer, you don't need to fear failure. Scientists thrive off failure—each failure brings them one step closer to the truth.

This isn't a new concept; I didn't invent the idea of self-experimentation. French philosopher Michel de Montaigne accumulated knowledge in his lifetime through self-experimentation, self-discovery, and observation. Ryan Holiday sums this up perfectly:

> Montaigne is a special philosophical figure because he didn't subscribe to one school of thought. Instead, he subscribed to all of them. He was willing to take bits and pieces from anywhere, as long as they had practical application to his life.[8]

I want you to adapt this same stream of thought. For every piece of information from this book that you decide to put into practice, acknowledge that it might not be the right fit for you. Self-observation is just as important as self-experimentation. All the ingredients are laid out, but you may have to combine different elements to get the end result you desire. You can pick out some different pieces and try again. Exploration and curiosity are both innate human qualities. If we're all able to get in touch with these qualities and reframe how we approach nutrition and training, we can develop long-lasting forms of motivation. Finding the right frame of mind is an important topic and something I touch on multiple times throughout this book. But for now, know that adopting an explorer mindset is how we can become active with our learning and turn ideas into action.

CHAPTER 2

Uncovering Sustainable Motivation

I just need a bit more motivation.
—EVERY SINGLE PERSON ON THIS EARTH

When I was a senior in high school, I desperately wanted to lose weight. No matter what I did and how extreme I dieted, the weight just wouldn't come off. I tried eating only salmon and egg whites for days on end, while getting my sweat on to the YouTube video *8 Minute Abs*[1] at least four to five days a week. In addition to the eight minutes of core torture, I also played rugby on my high school team, as well as competitive ice hockey. I was a pretty active kid.

I would go through these vicious cycles of starving myself and then binge eating. I would eat nothing but protein for an entire day and then come home from school and dig into two bowls of Reese's Puffs cereal, following that with a solid two-hour, teen-style nap. The food deprivation and the hamster wheel of shame and guilt caused me to develop an unhealthy relationship with food and a poor self-image.

I felt like I *had* to lose weight to be accepted. I experienced a lot of outside peer pressure that I think we can all relate to. Hearing secondhand murmurings from guys in my grade teasing me about my weight created an open wound that, to this day, sometimes stings. I wanted to eat what I wanted when I wanted, and my only driving force to lose weight at the time was the desire to fit in. In retrospect, I can easily pinpoint all the dieting mistakes I made, but at the time, I felt hopeless with my weight-loss efforts. I didn't understand how the other girls in my grade remained a size 2 while eating poutine (a Canadian delicacy of french fries with brown gravy and cheese curds) and M&M cookies every day at lunch. Teenage metabolisms— if you're unlucky enough to lose yours as a preteen, it can be a real bummer.

It wasn't until my second year of college that I had a "light bulb moment" and realized that being "thin" as the driving motivator to stay healthy probably wasn't going to be sustainable. I finally changed my outlook on health and wellness and found an approach to exercise and nutrition that worked for my body. While the fear of gaining the weight back was running the show for a while, I felt more empowered this time to stick with my plan. I wanted to change my relationship with my body and, at the same time, reap the other benefits of feeling more energized and confident in my own skin.

SELF-DETERMINATION THEORY

What I was experiencing, my friends, is the self-determination theory (SDT) in action. The self-determination theory framework was developed in the 1980s by two psychologists, Edward Deci and Richard Ryan. Their theory proposes that we, as humans, derive our motivation to take action and grow from harnessing three innate psychological needs: autonomy, relatedness, and competence.[2] In short, to harbor sustainable motivation while pursuing goals, we must have a healthy dose of these three needs. Let's break them down.

Autonomy is having control over our lives—choosing to participate and engage in activities for our own self-growth. Pursuing goals on an *intrinsic* level. When I started my fitness journey, I took ownership of the changes I wanted to see in my body composition, and I devised my own fitness routine and nutrition plan. I wanted the relationship with my body to change and took the necessary steps to get there. A great relationship with your body can come in many forms (not just in relation to weight): feeling confident in your skin, practicing self-love, owning all the amazing parts of your body, or just wanting to get into a healthier routine.

Relatedness is the way we feel connected or can relate to others. Fitness can help form connections, commonalities, and bonds among new people. When I started working out at the gym, I would go with friends or work out alongside other classmates. I later forged new friendships with people I'd never spoken to before by striking up conversations at the gym or in the change room.

Competence is the feeling of mastery when you develop a skill and feel confident in that discipline. As I mention in the introduction, I kicked off my new fitness regimen in my second year of college with a 22-minute interval treadmill workout. It was tough, but I designed the regimen so that it was still achievable—not so difficult that I couldn't stick with it. Over the course of a few weeks, I started getting better at my workout, slowly increasing the treadmill starting speed and, at the same time, staying on the harder levels a bit longer. By improving my speed, I started to feel more competent, which helped me develop a newfound passion for running.

So how was I able to make this new plan stick? What was different from when I tried to do the same in high school? It came down to this: In high school, I didn't want to change my existing diet and go to the gym. I didn't want to stop eating the foods I loved. I felt external pressure to fit into the pretty granular stereotype of what a cis woman should look like. I despised traditional cardio machines (elliptical, treadmills, bikes) and had zero interest in lifting weights. I played sports because I loved to (autonomy) and made good friends with my teammates (relatedness). I also did well at some sports (competence). In high school, I was named Rugby All-Star in the local paper and was later recruited to my university's rugby team.

In college, however, my interests started to change. I began moving away from team sports (hockey, rugby) and toward more individual activities, like running and weight lifting. Although I used to despise singular sports, in college I went from hating them to thinking they weren't so bad to fully enjoying them. As previously mentioned, I developed more commonalities among my classmates who also worked out at my university's gym (relatedness). I created my own training and nutrition plan that I researched extensively (autonomy). And I started getting good at my treadmill workout. I got stronger and began seeing palpable progress in my body composition (competence). However, only in retrospect can I conclude that the components of SDT were the catalyst in helping me sustain a consistent fitness regimen for years.

If we feel a loss of control or outward pressure to lose weight from friends, family, a partner, or society at large, we're less likely to stick to our commitments and goals over the long haul.[3] This makes sense. We don't like being told what to do. Rebellion is natural. We as humans thrive off making our own decisions and taking ownership of our lives. We gain confidence as we develop and successfully apply our skills. As natural explorers, we thrive from discovering answers on our own and are driven by our innate curiosity.

In American behavioral sustainability scientist Michelle Segar's book, *No Sweat*, she discusses how SDT can play a role in our relationship with exercise and affect our motivation to stick with it. She uses the example of someone taking up the activity of walking:

> An individual who feels controlled toward being physically active—say, being told that she must take a brisk forty-minute walk every day—would consider walking a *should*. To this person, walking is something she has to do in order to avoid a punishment, to comply with an external pressure. In contrast, an individual who feels autonomous towards walking decides to do it because she wants to do it in the ways that she chooses to do it.[4]

This person deeply values her own reasons for taking a walk, understands and acts on the benefits she gets from the activity, or simply experiences satisfaction from the process of being physically active.

We're more inclined to stick with an activity or exercise program if we deeply value or have a personal investment in the practice. However, if we feel like we *have to* or, in Segar's words, *should,* then the chances of following through are slim to none or we'll be stripped of enjoyment from the activity, and it will inevitably feel like a chore. Keep this in mind as you read the rest of the book.

INTRINSIC AND EXTRINSIC MOTIVATION

Another integral component of SDT is how intrinsic and extrinsic motivation and rewards play a role in achieving goals and the sustainability of processes. Extrinsic motivation is the drive to do something to gain an external reward. Wanting to run a marathon to achieve a medal or earn bragging rights is a prime example. Intrinsic motivation is the internal drive to do something that stems from our aspirations for self-growth. For example, the intrinsic motivation to run a marathon would be the desire to challenge yourself, to push farther than you thought possible with the end goal being improved performance—to become a better runner.

Intrinsic motivation is long-lasting and sustainable; extrinsic motivation is ephemeral. So which one is better to have when you set out on your fitness journey? Steve Magness and Brad Stulberg, creators of the popular blog *The Growth Equation*, recommend utilizing both types of motivation to help with consistency and the attainment of goals. However, extrinsic motivators should be used sparingly, just to drive immediate action.

No matter how far along you are in your fitness journey, you'll want to strike a balance between both forms of motivation but lean heavily toward intrinsic. Not to sound trite, but to persist, you do need to enjoy the process—find joy in and derive real pleasure from the activity itself.

You cannot stay consistent if you're relying solely on willpower and self-discipline, which are two finite and fast-depleting resources. Realizing that the work itself is the reward, and making an activity autotelic is a hallmark in sustainability.

Incorporating some external rewards along the way can help keep you engaged, but don't rely solely on them. Staying in that "high," whether it be earning that medal, winning a competition, or hitting a personal best on your 10K time, can prevent you from getting back to the actual work itself. It's great to celebrate your accomplishments, but set a boundary on when you'll take time off to rest, and then get back at it.

Here's how the SDT framework applies to my life and training: When I train and run every day to hit a specific weight-loss goal or pace, my workouts feel forced. My engagement is lacking, and training starts to feel like a chore. For I-don't-even-know-how-many years, I obsessively monitored my pace (especially on high-intensity efforts). If I made progress and hit a new personal best, then great, my efforts were paying off. If I didn't make progress, I'd feel a flurry of negative emotions: annoyed, deflated, and worthless. I realize these are extreme reactions, but it's the truth—I let my pace run the show.

When I reframe my training and remind myself of the more meaningful reasons why I train, I enjoy the activity exponentially more. For example, I use my training as a time to think through complex problems, disconnect from my phone and work, and soothe anxiety. The adrenaline and endorphins kicking in and sweat dripping down my face as I listen to my favorite electronic dance music (EDM) beats during a workout are euphoric. Running outdoors through trails, inhaling that piney smell, and feeling the sun shining on my face is cathartic. It's not weight loss or "staying fit" that has kept me running every day for the past four years; rather, the deeper meaning that I derive from the sport keeps me coming back day in and day out. Running is a time I carve out for myself every single day. This activity has given me grit, zeal, and perseverance, a mechanism I use to relieve my stress, clear my head, and subdue my stream of self-deprecating thoughts.

Challenge is one of my core values; I enjoy pushing myself to get better. That means signing up for races intermittently throughout the year. I like to work toward that personal best (intrinsic) and the medal and accolades (extrinsic). I also like to go through "cutting" phases—in which I track my calories and macronutrients (macros) to achieve visible physique results—and share my progress on social media (extrinsic). But at the same time, I use these activities as experiments, driven by a genuine curiosity (intrinsic) to see how specific diets or differing calorie/macro intakes track with my mood and energy levels. One of the biggest mistakes I've made is to focus too much on extrinsic forms of motivation to power my long-term goals. Don't get me wrong—the end result can feel really good, including crossing the finish line, getting a personal best time, the physiological endorphin boost post-run, and the dopamine hits from the laud I receive from sharing my accomplishments on social media. However it's the *doing* that brings about a meditative state that keeps me hooked.

BUILD YOUR MENTAL TOOLBOX

This sounds like a paradox, but seeking external sources of inspiration can help fuel your intrinsic motivation. For example, when you listen to people's anecdotal experiences or what drives them, it can serve as a foundation on which to build your own motivation.

Internal motivation requires upkeep, and on some days, it can be in short supply. So it's good to find a method that helps ground and remind you why you've set this goal in the first place. I keep an ongoing list of reasons why I love to run and train, which serves as a reference point that I can revert back to if I experience prolonged feelings of low motivation, fatigue, or procrastination. I call this my mental toolbox. I pack my arsenal with supportive quotations, inspirational stories, slivers of wisdom acquired through experience, personal stories of other athletes and how they conquered adversity, or other random and helpful thoughts I can pull from to light a fire under me. You can keep this archive in any form you like. I like to store it digitally in my journaling app, Day One. Best-selling author Ryan Holiday keeps a commonplace book and stores his ideas on index cards. When famous choreographer Twyla Tharp starts a new project, she stores photos, video files, newspaper clippings, and other inspiration in a new box. Whatever your method, digital or analog, keeping these reminders can be a strong driving force behind staying motivated.

The following are examples of how I apply forms of motivation to my daily runs and how I derive deeper meaning from my running:

- I will use today's outdoor run to listen to an audiobook and learn something new.

- On today's longer run, I will plug in a psychological thriller audio-book, which I always find relaxing and enjoyable.

- I will not listen to anything today—I'm faced with a difficult problem, and I need this time to disconnect and think through some solutions.

- I'm feeling debilitating anxiety tonight, so I'm going to go for a light jog (which always makes me feel better).

- I will use today's run to percolate on a book I just read, a blog post idea I'm formulating, or the content for a social media post.

Get into the habit of jotting down how your training makes you *feel.* You may see recurring answers, but you might also be surprised to find new and exciting ways your training can bring more meaning to your life.

THE LONG GAME

It took me weeks of consistent effort in my workouts and diet to start seeing small changes in my body. It took me three years of training and slowly building up mileage to run my first half marathon. I took a couple more years to build up the endurance (and courage) to run my first marathon. After 10 long years I finally saw the muscle definition I wanted. The point is that when it comes to fitness, patience is critical. Fat loss, muscle gain, body transformations, and most importantly, mind shifts, do not happen overnight. They are a result of consistent work over prolonged periods of time.

I wrote this book for those who want to shift their relationship with their body, see physical transformations in their body, or perhaps just find a sustainable nutrition and workout plan that works for them. To find success, I think it's more important to equip yourself mentally and find a nutrition and training plan that you enjoy—a plan that's realistic and doesn't require an inordinate amount of willpower every day to complete. You can't feel ongoing deprivation or relate training with torture. If you do, it's going to be one hell of a journey.

We must learn to fall in love with the process. This piece of wisdom has been repeated tirelessly; however, it holds true. To be a contender in the long game of fitness, you need to find joy in the exercises you're doing and the food you're eating. That's not to say that you're going to want to exercise every day. Rarely do I spring out of bed and want to work out with vigor and enthusiasm. Even after 14 years of consistent running and training, I still feel resistance. Some days are worse than others, but I know that I will always feel better if I train. The payoff is worth exerting the effort.

Our minds are powerful and sometimes predictable instruments. If you equate exercise with hell and torture, then—spoiler alert—it will be hell and torture. The first step is to acknowledge where you are and decide where you want to be. Not just for the next few months as you gear up for beach season. What kind of relationship with exercise do you want in the long term? My training and running time is my opportunity to decompress, de-stress, and jam to whatever audio I'm feeling that day. My daily runs are also when my mental health becomes my only priority. I love the burn after lifting heavy weights and exhausting my muscles.

When it comes to getting "fit"—whatever that means and looks like for you—the tortoise will always win. The hare will experience burnout, yo-yo dieting, and the many frustrations and discouragement that accompany an inability to stick to an unsustainable commitment. Michelle Segar calls the epidemic of starting-quitting-starting-quitting the "vicious cycle of failure."[5] To avoid this, you need to enjoy your training and nutrition plan, and set realistic goals and commitment levels based on your current lifestyle. Most importantly, know that intrinsic motivation and incorporating autonomy, relatedness, and competence are keys for sustaining a fitness regimen.

CHAPTER 3

Developing Lifelong Habits

Habits matter because they help you become the person you wish to be. They are the channel to which you develop the deepest beliefs about yourself.

—JAMES CLEAR, *Atomic Habits*

First off, let me just say that I am not an expert on habit formation; nor do I pretend to be. I am not Charles Duhigg or James Clear, although a gal can dream. Duhigg, author of the *New York Times* best-selling book *The Power of Habit*, and James Clear, author of the *New York Times* best seller *Atomic Habits* (over 2 million copies sold) have both written amazing literature. Duhigg and Clear provide a much stronger narrative around this topic than I could ever offer. However, I think it's important to briefly summarize important theoretical frameworks on how habits work and how we can alter components of the habit loop to help us build and sustain lifelong practices in the areas of fitness and nutrition. I add some unique perspectives on the topic where I can.

Habits form the foundational backbone of who we are. They're an automatic response from a neurological feedback loop and can be positive or negative. For a habit to be established and remembered by the brain, we need to cycle through the habit loop numerous times. It goes like this:

Cue → Action → Reward → Cue → Action → Reward

Repeat forever

Let's break down each of these three components further:

Step 1: Cue. A cue, or trigger, tells your mind to initiate an action. Time- and location-based cues are the most common, but a preceding event or some sort of emotion or internal feeling can also be a cue. For example, your alarm goes off and you hit "brew" on the coffee maker; you walk into the kitchen, which is your cue to grab a snack; or the clock strikes noon, signaling time for lunch.

Step 2: Action. This is the response to the cue that you perform to get some form of a reward. Again, your motivation to take action is an important factor. If the action is too hard or, as Clear writes, "requires more physical or mental effort than you're willing to expend, then you won't do it."[1] This is the last step before you reach the finish line to that reward, so it better be worth it if you are going to take any necessary action.

Step 3: Reward. The reward needs to satiate us and train our minds to either repeat the habit or *not* repeat the habit. After the reward is obtained, the habit loop closes and starts from the beginning again. If the reward is satisfying, we're more likely to repeat a behavior; if it sucks, well, we probably won't stick with it. A hard cardio session followed by a big reward of a plate of spinach, for example. No, thanks.

I discuss some strategies shortly on optimizing each of the habit-loop components to build and sustain healthy habits and, more importantly, to enjoy them. To make the loop strong and sturdy, we need to make sure the cue is evident in our environment, the action is as easy and as close to the reward as possible, and the reward is satisfying.

The previous chapter discusses how self-determination theory's motivational groundwork of autonomy, competence, and relatedness drives us to accomplish our goals. It also discusses how uncovering deeper meaning and intrinsic rewards in your training is integral to sustaining a regimen. Let's look at some practical applications of this theoretical framework when it comes to building sustainable habits.

OPTIMIZING THE HABIT LOOP FOR YOUR TRAINING

Cue

Cues all start with awareness. We need to either be aware of the cue already, which is particularly important when it comes to bad habits, or create one from scratch. All in all, a cue needs to be obvious in our environment. There's a principle in habit formation called *implementation intention*, which increases the likelihood that you'll perform the action required in the habit loop. Setting our intentions, such as when and where we'll work out, can exponentially increase our likelihood of completing a desired action.

The first thing you need to do is write those intentions down. Write them down. No, seriously, *write them down*. I repeat this because I can't stress its importance enough, and I'm also trying to annoy you (just kidding!). Make sure to include the time and day when you will train and the workout you plan on doing, which is a critical component when trying to optimize cues.

I try and stick to 9:00 a.m. every day to do my workouts. The timing is a bit more malleable on weekends because I like to sleep in, wake up slowly, and read or work on creative projects. But during the week, I'm pretty meticulous with my schedule and regimen. If you're not able to stick to a regularly scheduled time, pick another time or come up with a contingency plan. Sometimes I have client meetings in other time zones and need to do early morning calls. It screws with my schedule, but I just work around it and start my workout either before or immediately after a meeting. It's good to have a set routine, but it's also important to realize that life happens. Things don't always go according to plan every day, so it's essential to give yourself the flexibility to work around any curveballs. Be agile and choose an alternative time. With my running, I don't give myself a choice. I run every day, whether it's on the treadmill or outdoors, which is mainly dependent on the weather (hello, we have −15°F Canadian winters here) and my accessibility to a treadmill. I decide the day before where I'll run.

I assign a particular body part to each weekday for exercising that specific group of muscles. This helps me alleviate some of the pre-routine questioning of what I'm going to do for each workout. For example, Monday is upper-body pull (biceps/traps/back), Tuesday is core, Wednesday is upper-body push (shoulders/chest/triceps), and so on.

Environment is an important cue as well. As I write this, we're still in the midst of the COVID-19 pandemic, so I've been working out at home more frequently. I prefer the gym (I like all the fancy equipment, the community aspect, and the nice lineup of dumbbell options). However, if you prefer to work out from home or are forced to because gyms are closed, it's important to carve out a little space in your home that can be your exercise cave. Preferably, this would be in a different room from where you work and chill, but if that's not an option, then make a little exercise corner for yourself. When I'm in my workout space or in my parents' basement, for example, my brain switches into workout mode. When I'm sitting at my desk, I'm in work mode. I've struggled with switching from work to home life over the years, but separating these spaces in my home has helped trigger desired behaviors.

Action

The physical movement or action is the most challenging part of a workout and where most of us fail. The first few minutes of my workouts are always the worst, but once I'm in the groove, my workouts take a turn toward the enjoyable. Like every other human on this planet, I procrastinate. I have bad days, when I experience low energy and struggle to complete my workouts. I have low to empty willpower reserves. However, there are a few tricks I've learned over the years that make action a bit easier and can help you trick yourself into being excited for your workout.

It all starts with a workout ritual. We often talk about the power and effectiveness of routines, but when it comes to motivation, the idea of "rituals" isn't as ubiquitous. Our everyday activities and routines can be monotonous and boring. When perceived as a chore, they can cause what Steven Pressfield calls "the Resistance"[2]—routines become something we have to do, instead of something we want to do, and then we resist.

Twyla Tharp is one of America's greatest choreographers, with more than 130 dances under her belt. Not only is she prolific in her craft, but she is also well known for her consistent and almost religious workout ritual:

> I wake up at 5:30 A.M., put on my workout clothes, my leg warmers, my sweatshirts, and my hat. I walk outside my Manhattan home, hail a taxi, and tell the driver to take me to the Pumping Iron gym . . . where I work out for two hours. The ritual is not the stretching and weight training I put my body through each morning at the gym: the ritual is the cab. The moment I tell the driver where to go I have completed the ritual.[3]

A habit is an automatic behavior, a routine requires more effort and intention to sustain, and a ritual is more of a mental practice to put you in a good headspace. Rituals traditionally have a spiritual or religious connotation but can be applied to the mundane, everyday routines to give us more purpose and joy behind a seemingly boring activity. Rituals turn the arduous into the exciting, the mundane into the fun, the repetitive into the fresh and new.

We've all heard stories of athletes who have their own idiosyncratic pre-game rituals. Of course, you may already have one yourself. Sleeping in your workout clothes, listening to your pump-up music, and having your pre-gym coffee are all examples of small—but effective—routines.

If you work out in the morning, start your ritual the night before. Every night before I go to bed, I get the coffee ready to go and lay out the gym clothes I'm going to wear. Immediately upon waking up, I put on my gym clothes and make my bed. I need at least an hour or two to wake up my brain by reading, writing, and getting my coffee on before I start my workout. At 8:45 a.m., I put my running shoes on, brush my teeth, stick in my headphones, ramp up some beats, and mix my pre-workout drink. By 9:00, I'm primed and ready to start. I try to minimize any roadblocks that keep me from beginning my workout. I always start easy: a bit of muscular endurance work, or if I'm doing cardio first, I'll run the first kilometer or so at an easy, steady-state pace. The key is to make your workout ritual as easy and manageable as possible. Mornings aren't easy for everyone.

On bad days, when procrastination kicks in and the thought of working out is the last thing I feel like doing, I play a few games with my mind to get me in the zone. The biggest one is telling myself I can run fewer miles today, focus on low intensity, or only do one body part (such as my back). If I had planned to get in a high-mileage day (20+ kilometers/13 miles), I will some-times break up the run into two workouts: a 7-mile run in the morning and a 6.1-mile run in the evening, for instance. Some people tell themselves that they "will work out for *only* 20 minutes." Sounds a hell of a lot better than 1 hour. Go into the workout with a smaller goal, and if, and only if, you feel like it, then go longer.

The takeaway in the action or response stage is to try and figure out how to make starting your training as easy as possible. Creating a workout ritual and convincing yourself that you can make it shorter if you're not *feeling it* can be powerful motivators to get you to move. Also, remember that every-thing counts. Even a 5- or 10-minute run is always better than no run at all. It doesn't need to be all or nothing.

Reward

The rewards are the fun part, and this is where I like to experiment. Here's the thing about rewards: they are deeply individual. Rewards come in all shapes and sizes, in all different experiences and circumstances. They are also so much more satisfying if we earn them. For example, earning a million dollars through sheer hard work is more satisfying than winning a million dollars in the lottery. Although I wouldn't say no to the latter.

Remember that rewards can be intrinsic or extrinsic. If a reward is external (such as weight loss), keep in mind that changes in your body don't happen overnight. That's why intrinsic rewards are so, so important and integral to building an exercise habit and sustaining it. We get the immediate high of endorphins and feel good, and any negative feelings we're carrying—whether they're from a bad work experience, relationship troubles, or realizing we're officially out of popcorn—begin to dissipate.

Dr. Alison Phillips, assistant researcher of psychology at Iowa State University, and colleagues conducted a study and found that it takes more than just a cue to stick with an exercise routine. They suggest that the combination of a cue and an intrinsic reward drives us to create habits and stick with them.[4] A morning alarm clock or a predetermined time that we schedule an action isn't enough. We need to uncover that deeper meaning for sustainability. As with the mental toolbox, every time you finish a workout and discover a new benefit you haven't experienced before, jot it down, read it over, and remember it. These intrinsic motivators are integral to helping us form a habit and, more importantly, sticking with it for the long run.

When you're figuring out your rewards, put on your curiosity cap and get experimenting. The goal is to make your workouts more enjoyable by peppering them with intermittent pleasures and desirable actions.

I like to mix in rewards intermittently throughout my training and then give myself a big reward at the end, which can be extrinsic or intrinsic. That way, I'm closing the action-reward loop sooner. I'm taking action and getting a reward quickly, which keeps me coming back for more and helps me sustain longer workouts (1.5–2 hours).

The first reward I get is before I even start my workout. Immediately after putting on my running shoes, I get to mix my intra-workout drink, a delicious blend of BCAAs[5] and creatine that's bursting with sour peach–flavored deliciousness. Next, I use a gigantic water jug, which is fittingly called "Mammoth Mug," and sip on it between my sets.

Between my strength and cardio sessions, I'll usually take a little break and give myself a dopamine reward. I'll check my email, hop on social media for a sec, or reply to a text message. Unless I'm in a rush, I like to give myself a 5-minute break to decompress before moving on to the next phase of my workout.

Going to the gym with a partner? Why don't you give each other a kiss between sets? I mean, this might require a specific degree of coordination, but it makes working out a lot more fun (and cute)!

Stop and walk between intervals. When you're doing a hard workout, the feeling of walking immediately afterward will provide an instantaneous reward of relief. Give yourself an opportunity to walk a bit between intervals or stretch out your muscles between sets.

A powerful reward at the end of your workout might be to share it on social media, which can provide a huge dopamine hit. If it's a run, you can use an app like MapMyRun (UA), Strava, or NRC (Nike). While this may be annoying for some, I love seeing other people's workouts fill up my feed— I find it inspiring. Sharing details of my daily runs during the #RUN70 challenge also helped build an online community because people enjoyed following along. Their supportive messages were a catalyst in pushing me forward throughout the challenge—especially on rough days. However, I would be remiss not to warn that too much sharing on social media and relying on accolades from others to fuel motivation can have a pernicious effect. If the laud and cheers don't arrive, we may get discouraged. And even if they do, we may develop an insatiable appetite for them that can only be filled with more likes and more comments. Just be wary of sharing your efforts for egocentric reasons; as previously mentioned, allowing your ego to drive your fitness journey is not sustainable.

Another rewards tactic you could try is *temptation bundling*, a concept coined by behavioral economist Katherine L. Milkman. The idea is to increase your likelihood of exercising by pairing an undesired behavior with a desired one. Milkman and colleagues conducted a study that they hilariously named "Holding the Hunger Games Hostage at the Gym: An Evaluation of Temptation Bundling," to see if they could increase exercise rates using people's favorite audiobooks.[6]

In the first group, the researchers gave people who wanted to exercise an iPod loaded with four audiobooks of their choosing that they could listen to *only* at the gym during their workouts. Participants had to turn in their iPods after workouts, and they couldn't listen to the audiobooks until they returned to the gym. Temptation bundling was suggested and enforced.

The researchers gave the second group an iPod containing four favorite novels, but the participants were told they could access the books whenever they wanted to. They were also told about the benefits of temptation bundling and encouraged to listen only while exercising, but it wasn't enforced.

A third control group was given a Barnes and Noble gift card in the monetary equivalent of four audiobooks and was educated on the importance of exercise on their health during the study intake period.

Over the first seven-week period, Milkman and colleagues saw gym attendance for the first group increase by 51%; it increased by 44% in the second group and 42% in the control group. But—and this is a big but—the study also saw a significant decline in gym attendance over the Thanksgiving holiday, and the benefits of temptation bundling began to taper off. Following the Thanksgiving break, gym attendance and weekly minutes exercised declined significantly. Another critical variable to mention is that this program worked only for those who enjoyed listening to audiobooks while working out. In short, you need to enjoy the reward for it to be effective—spinach just ain't going to cut it (or maybe it will if you're into that).

Psychological thrillers are my guilty pleasure, and I would say that the *Hunger Games* series is part of my "addictive books" lineup. During my #RUN70 challenge, I would let myself listen to these novels only during longer runs. Once I started the run, I'd press Play. Once it was over, I'd hit Pause. This was particularly effective when I approached the climax in the story that was met with an abrupt end when I finished my run. I couldn't wait to lace up my running shoes the next day and dive back into my book!

Here's another one: Do you ever find new music that you're obsessed with and play on repeat a million times? Even if you hit the jackpot on Spotify's Release Radar, only let yourself listen to that song or song(s) when you're training and no other times of the day. Then, when you start your workout, give yourself an immediate reward of listening to that song or song(s). Repeat as many times as you want, but then stop when you're done.

If you are going to use temptation bundling, just be aware that you do need to still exert some self-control. The tool is a great way to kick off a habit and stick with it for a bit, but it doesn't last forever. You will still need to find intrinsic motivation to sustain your efforts over the long haul.

Rewards are truly endless. Get creative with yours, and conduct ongoing experiments. Incorporate several rewards throughout your training (and more toward the beginning to get you going), and you'll be more inclined to not only start your workout but also keep at it for an extended period of time.

30-DAY CHALLENGES

The idea behind building a habit in 30 days is old news, with study after study showing varying results on the number of days it really takes to build a habit. For example, one study showed an average of 66 days to reach automaticity (where habits become automatic behaviors), with a big disparity among participants—some took only 8 days, while others took up to 200 days to form a habit.[7] While you may not be able to build a sustainable habit over a 30-day timeline, devising a challenge for approximately one month is a great way to dip your toe into a new change rather than diving in headfirst.

One of the most popular bloggers on self-development, Steve Pavlina, regularly incorporates 30-day or even 365-day challenges to explore a lifestyle change or develop a skill. Pavlina experimented with veganism back in the 1990s, which was the impetus behind his decision to become fully vegan. In 2020, he wrote and published a blog post every day for 365 days. In 2021, he set a goal to eat only raw foods for 365 days. While Pavlina's willpower is stronger than many people's, he's a big proponent of the explorer mindset (discussed in Chapter 1), which is about finding out your own truth through experimentation.

The 10-kilometers-per-day challenge I did in January 2017 (it was 31 days actually, but close enough) changed the trajectory of my life. Clearly, I'm a big fan of the format. I've conducted 30-day challenges with blog writing, veganism, vegetarianism, sobriety, meditation, and other changes I wanted to further explore. I even created a #RUN30 Consecutive Running Challenge on my blog to provide tools and tips for other runners who want to challenge themselves to run a set distance every day for 30 days straight.

While 30 days may seem like a lot, the consistency can help a habit form or at least give you peace of mind on whether this is an activity you want to pursue or incorporate into your lifestyle.

As you may have noticed by now, I'm a big proponent of running personal experiments throughout the year, and I encourage you to do the same. This mentality is also important (as you'll see when we get to nutrition and training) when testing out different macro splits, figuring out your maintenance calories, and incorporating different training plans.

You may decide to drop a particular nutrition plan or exercise regimen after the 30 days are up, or you may find that you want to stick with it. Or you might want to incorporate bits and pieces that you enjoyed and toss aside the others. Not only are you repeating the desired behavior, but you also are learning to alter activities in your life to make time for you.

One last thing to note about 30-day challenges is that they can be even more powerful and meaningful if you share them with the world. It will keep you accountable and inspire others—an incredible side effect of taking on a self-growth experiment. Regardless of whether you keep that change in your life, I can almost guarantee that your life will be altered in one way or another. You will gain new perspectives, develop more self-discipline, and feel confident that you are able to stick to a commitment you set for yourself.

OPTIMIZING THE HABIT LOOP FOR YOUR DIET

When the COVID-19 pandemic began, I moved in temporarily with my parents. For a few days, I casually observed what my mom ate in a day and noticed that her protein intake was really low, based on her current weight. I asked if she wanted some help with getting her daily protein intake up and she did. So together we created a cue for her—a reminder to try to incorporate more protein in her diet—which we both agreed was a great way to achieve her daily protein goals. I proposed an idea of a protein guide to stick on the fridge, and she was game.[8]

The guide was broken out by animal products, grains, vegetables and fruit, condiments and seasonings, and nuts and nut butters. I listed all the foods my mom included in her diet, as well as some new items she was willing to try. Each item included the average serving size, and I placed my food scale on the counter and showed my mom how to use it. I also put a "daily protein intake" goal for her on the fridge right underneath the guide, so it functioned as a constant reminder.

Almost immediately, my mom's protein intake increased from around 60 g per day to well over 100 g. She found it fun adding up her protein points and hitting her goals. We also made some swaps. My mom loves chocolate or baked goods mid-afternoon and is obsessed with caramel (the lady's got fine taste). I bought her some chocolate caramel peanut protein bars with only 1 g of sugar and 20 g of protein to eat instead. I asked her what she liked about the new system, and she said she was better informed about her choices. She was surprised to learn that adding four tablespoons of tzatziki to her crackers and cheese snack gave her an extra 10 g of protein! She felt good because she was eating healthier; protein is more satiating than carbs and fat, so when she increased her protein, she wasn't eating as much food in general during the day.

My mom didn't remove any foods from her diet besides the desserts she swapped for the protein bar, but the bar is so yummy that she didn't feel deprived at all. I also didn't force her into this experiment. She wanted to get more protein and was autonomous about the decision. If my mom had felt resentful or like it was forced on her (remember our good ol' friend SDT), I can guarantee she wouldn't have stuck with it, which is a feeling many people can relate to.

If you want to break a bad eating habit, you need to be aware of the cue or trigger that's causing the behavior. If you want to develop better eating habits, create an obvious trigger to remind you to make healthier choices. Eliminating all the foods you love isn't sustainable; it's deprivation. I expand more on food swaps and understanding your own calorie and macro needs in Part II, so stay tuned.

MAINTAINING YOUR HABITS

Research shows that when starting a new habit, self-discipline is needed. In the long term, building on that habit starts to get easier to maintain; this holds true once we start to master the habit and it delivers ongoing intrinsic rewards.

Something that is rarely talked about in the realm of habits is the need for self-compassion. In other words, be easy on yourself if you slip up, in whatever capacity that might be. If you struggle with the upkeep of commitments you've set for yourself, then you might be met with a side of guilt and shame, which inevitably leads to a hit to your self-esteem. I've been there too many times to count, and a shortage of self-compassion can also increase undesired behaviors (e.g., eat a bit of ice cream, feel terrible for breaking your commitments or ruining your diet, and then end up consuming the whole tub while you are fueled by emotional eating).

Remind yourself that you will fall off the path. You will have hiccups. We all do. If you feel that you've fallen off the horse and failed one day, get back in the saddle tomorrow. If you're facing roadblocks every day, try to understand the root of the problem. Are you writing down a plan? Are your workouts too hard, too often? Are you doing the wrong kind of workouts (i.e., activities you don't enjoy)? Do the rewards suck? Try to experiment with different parts of the habit loop to settle on a plan that works for you.

Think of it like this: Scientists don't chastise themselves if their hypotheses are proven wrong. Each failed experiment is one step closer to the truth. Every time you fail to uphold your commitments to yourself, you are one step closer to finding a plan that works for you. So don't be afraid of the "f" word; as long as you learn from it and give yourself some loving, then you're doing just fine, my friend.

CHAPTER 4

Setting Your Fitness Goals

I f you're getting antsy to move on to the nutrition and training sections, I feel ya. But I promise that this chapter is a worthwhile topic to discuss and will make your fitness journey more enjoyable, easier, fun, and most importantly, sustainable. Remember that my goal with this book is to set you up for success over the *long term*. I want you to not only achieve your aesthetic fitness goals but also develop a consistent regimen, find deeper (intrinsic) meaning in your training, and draw on the many benefits of fitness, which can be applied to other facets of your life.

WHY MOST PEOPLE FAIL TO ACHIEVE THEIR FITNESS GOALS

Most people who set fitness goals and New Year's resolutions flounder after the first few months, and even sometimes mere weeks after the outset of the goal. I think it's become ubiquitous at this point. Once the initial enthusiasm of a fitness goal wears off, we're just left with the hard work. We approach fitness with large, grandiose plans to transform our body composition, go hard at the gym, and stick to a rigorous diet for a week or two. Then when we don't see results right away, we quit. Statistics vary on when the drop-off occurs, but it's usually within the first couple of months after setting the initial goal. According to a study conducted by the *Journal of Clinical Psychology*, as the year progresses and the drop-off rate continues to skyrocket, only 8% of people actually stick to the goals they set at the beginning of the year.[1]

But *why?*

The following are some of the most common reasons many people do not achieve their goals:

- Setting goals that lack personal meaning with too much emphasis on the extrinsic (or egocentric)

- Choosing vague or immeasurable goals (e.g., "lose weight")

- Setting unrealistic goals with high expectations of short-term success

- Setting lofty, long-term goals without breaking them down into smaller, more digestible milestones

- Going too hard at the outset and burning out

- Failing to see the scale move in the desired direction

And the list of reasons goes on, of course.

THE GOALS DEBATE

First, let's clarify what goals are. A goal is the object of a person's ambition or effort; it's an aim or desired result. When we think of fitness goals, for instance, we may immediately think "lose 10 pounds" or "gain 10 pounds of lean mass" or "achieve 10% body fat percentage" or "get a six pack." However, a goal also indicates an end point, a journey with a final destination, so it could be a single accomplishment (running a marathon) or hitting a specific number on the scale (body fat percentage, ideal weight, and so on).

The idea behind setting goals is a point of contention among productivity, habit, and fitness experts alike. There's much debate on whether you should even set goals at all (specifically metrics-based or numerical goals). "Goals should be an end-point, a wrap-up," writes productivity expert and author of *The Productivity Project*, Chris Bailey.[2]

As habit expert James Clear explains, we should focus more on systems as the alternative. Clear writes, "True long-term thinking is goal-less thinking. It's not about any single accomplishment. It is about the cycle of endless refinement and continuous improvement. Ultimately, it is your commitment to the process that will determine your progress."[3] In a similar vein, Bailey suggests focusing on our projects and habits instead. Brad Stulberg, performance coach and author of *The Practice of Groundedness*, says that we should focus on principles instead of goals—"things like health, creativity, movement, intellect, curiosity, and presence."[4]

None of these experts are telling us to fully neglect goals and their role, but they all agree that goals should take a back seat. The primary focus instead should be on figuring out and focusing on the process, habits, or principles we want to incorporate into our lives in the long term. By focusing on the process or "systems," we're better equipped to handle adversity and setbacks and more likely to succeed in attaining our actual goal.

MY FAILURES WITH GOAL SETTING

I would agree with the experts, and while I don't think setting goals is bad per se, I think there's a right and wrong way to set them. My biggest failures mainly stemmed from a lack of meaning behind the goals I set and no real endpoint or performance indicator that I was moving in the right direction. Some of my goals were too rigid and egocentric (revolved heavily around external validation). One of the shallower goals I've had over the years, for instance, was to obtain the elusive six-pack abs look. Naively, I worked out my core almost every day, and when I didn't see abs form after a few weeks of intense effort, I'd stop doing ab work altogether. This persisted for years: short bursts of hard effort, quick burnout, no results, quit, then repeat. I finally saw results when I let go of the goal of obtaining visible abs and, instead, focused on strengthening my core to improve my running and posture and stuck to my workout plan. I achieved these results by training core only two times per week while adhering to the principles of progressive overload. Then, over time, my abdominal muscles eventually began to creep to the surface. It took about a year and a half of consistent training to kind of see them and two years for them to become noticeable. After that, I had to trust the process and found more meaning than just having six-pack abs for vanity purposes. Simply setting an arbitrary numerical weight-loss goal or using fitness only as a means to boost sex appeal—to look ripped or "swole," lean, or jacked—is likely going to be a weak long-term frame, one that will eventually fizzle out over time, causing sporadic workouts, yoyo-dieting, and a dysfunctional relationship to fitness.

Another common issue that can arise is setting goals that are too restrictive, which may force ourselves into a rigid box, thus sparking all sorts of problems. If we fall off or "cheat" even slightly because, well, life happens, we chastise ourselves, and our self-confidence takes a blow for failing to stick with our commitments. There's also a cyclical component worth noting. Say we set the common goal to lose 10 pounds. We follow a strict eating and training plan and once we hit our goal, we pat ourselves on the back, give ourselves whatever reward we want, and then slowly but surely, we revert back to our old habits. The weight creeps up again and a few months later we're thinking, *Hmmm, I should probably lose 10 pounds*. The cycle repeats on and on—a hamster wheel of self-deprecation and not making any real progress over the long run. Sound familiar? I've certainly been there. When it comes to body recomposition goals, striving to hit a certain metric or aesthetic look can be distressful. Unless you're a bodybuilder or physique athlete, focusing and obsessing over metrics can be destructive and actually sabotage your efforts.

Having aesthetic goals is important and also fun. We're human. We love vanity. Having a body we feel confident in (whatever that looks like for you) and feeling physically strong improve our self-confidence. In the pursuance of our goals and challenges, we develop and strengthen our self-discipline, translating into gains in other areas of our lives.

When it comes to fitness, however, a specific goal can't be the only thing we strive for. There may also be a time when the goal no longer serves you. You may reach your body recomposition goals and then think, *Now what?*

This exact scenario happened to me more recently when I hit a bit of a ceiling with my body recomposition. I noticed changes becoming increasingly incremental, which forced me to look inward and find deeper meaning in my training to keep up my consistent routine.

Furthermore, if you don't enjoy the activity and find an ounce of pleasure in the process, the willpower tank will run dry and your engine will seize. Quitting will be the most likely scenario.

If we focus on the process instead, showing up and doing the best we can, we're much more likely to succeed over the long term. To summarize, the process should be the focal point, and, yes, we should set goals—they give us a target to move toward—but remember that they should be interpreted as an endpoint. Running a marathon is a great goal, but once you cross the finish line, it's done. When it comes to losing weight, building muscles, or any sort of physique goals, ask yourself this: Once you achieve this goal, are you done? Likely not, which leads me to discuss the importance of goal setting.

TIPS ON SETTING GOALS YOU'LL ACTUALLY STICK WITH

What kind of role do you want fitness to play in your life? How does training make you feel? Why do you want to make these changes?

Write out a list of your fitness training goals and observe whether most of your reasons are focused on the external (e.g., to look hot, to attract a partner, to take smokin' hot photos for the 'gram, etc.). I'm going to bet that your efforts probably won't be sustainable or they'll feel forced. On the other hand, if you focus on setting goals based on how they make you *feel* and uncover more intrinsic reasons (as outlined in the SDT theory), you're more likely to achieve your goals and remain consistent over time. For example, my goals are to obtain more energy so I can show up more in my relationships and work, to help with my posture, and to improve my technique at the gym and form in my running (competency).

When choosing goals, sports psychologists recommend the following framework that involves breaking out our goals by *outcome*, *performance*, and *process*:

- *Outcome:* This is the long-term end result.

- *Performance:* What are your key performance indicators (KPIs)? What is the measurable standard?[5]

- *Process:* How are you going to get there? What does your commitment level look like?

Instead of setting a numerical goal, I like to set timed experiments or 30-day challenges with the changes I want to make. The results materialize from the process.

VIA NEGATIVA: THE ART AND EFFECTIVENESS OF SUBTRACTION

Most people set goals with addition in mind, which include adding new habits, exercising more, eating more vegetables, adding a new diet plan. However, developing new habits and creating automaticity require significant self-discipline, energy, and time to foster. An easier and sometimes neglected route to goal setting is the art of subtraction, which can be defined as *via negativa*. This term stems from a method of theological thinking (used most commonly in Christian theology) to describe what God *is* by systematically removing what God *is not*. The term was popularized and further elucidated by Nassim Nicholas Taleb in his best-selling book *Antifragile*. Taleb writes, "The greatest—and most robust—contribution to knowledge consists in removing what we think is wrong—subtractive epistemology."[6] In practice, the "less-is-more idea"[7] can be more effective than addition in helping us attain our goals; you may find that removing bad habits is easier than adding positive ones.

For instance, to lose fat, you should focus on creating a caloric deficit—the removal of daily calories. Lifting weights—doing fewer reps with higher weight—can help you build more muscle. Removing alcohol from your diet will give you more energy and money to pursue more meaningful and fulfilling goals. Doing intervals (running for less time in faster increments) will improve your running economy, VO2 max, and make you a faster runner.

In 2021, two-thirds of the fitness-related goals I set were focused on *via negativa* and included *removing* meat from my diet by eating vegetarian for 30 consecutive days and abstaining from drinking any alcohol for six months. In addition, I also set the goal of hitting the four-year mark of running an average of 10 kilometers per day consecutively (which I hit in May 2021). The following framework breaks down the goals I set during my 30-day vegetarian challenge:

- *Outcome:* Eat only vegetarian for 30 consecutive days, and write a blog post about the experience.

- *Performance:* Remove meat for 30 days, journal about my energy levels and mood once per week, and use the photo journaling method to track any changes to my body composition over the course of the month.

- *Process:* Research plant-based protein and protein combinations to ensure I get all nine essential amino acids every day, learn new vegan and vegetarian recipes to incorporate into my diet, and buy any foods to support my new nutrition plan.

APPROACHING GOALS FROM A PLACE OF CURIOSITY

Curiosity is a mental framing (or intrinsic motivation) that has provided me with strong motivation to fuel my creative work. Lately, I've been testing this framing in setting my training and nutrition goals as well. Since human beings are innately curious, why not test this framework when setting our fitness goals? While this is a bit of an unconventional approach to fitness, this framing has helped me persist and complete the challenges and goals I've set for myself. I encourage you to get creative with your approach as well. Akin to a scientist, I positioned the 30-day vegetarian challenge as more of an experiment with some questions fueled by my own innate curiosity: How would this diet impact my running and training performance? How would this affect my body composition? Would I be able to get enough protein to support muscle growth? How would this diet impact my mood and energy levels?

After reading plant-based athlete Rich Roll's *Finding Ultra* and Scott Jurek's *Eat and Run*, I was part inspired and part curious to explore the vegetarian and vegan lifestyle. Curiosity gave me enough motivation to not only formulate the challenge but also acquire the necessary knowledge to help me succeed. The same goes for my six-month alcohol-free challenge; I was curious about how taking a prolonged break from alcohol would affect my body composition and mental health. So, reader, regarding fitness and nutrition, I ask you this: *What are you curious about?*

MAPPING OUT YOUR GOALS

In the subsequent training and nutrition parts of the book, I help you acquire the necessary knowledge to make your aesthetic goals a reality. More importantly, I teach you some tactics I've learned over the years to help you enjoy both your nutrition and training and make them sustainable. I did not write this book for anyone interested in immediate results, drastic changes, or "hacks." I wrote it for anyone who is all in on committing themselves to the process, which means acquiring the necessary knowledge and skills to get there.

You don't have to have all the answers right away, so don't worry. As you progress through your fitness journey and find the activities you really enjoy, you can incorporate new and more meaningful reasons to keep up your routine. For now, though, I want to give you two important warnings:

1. Unless training for a physique/bodybuilding show, be careful tracking metrics as key performance indicators, specifically the number that's showing up on the scale. Your weight never tells the whole story, and obsessing about the numbers can be discouraging and demotivating (more on this soon).

2. The cyclical nature of dieting and weight loss is a trap we don't want to fall into. Try to keep in mind a longer-term vision for yourself and how you want fitness and nutrition to play a role. What do you want your life to look like 5, 10, 20, or 30 years down the road?

Focus on your own competence, your own mastery, and your own fitness journey. You have no idea when or how other people started out on their journey and honestly, who really cares? Egocentric people who constantly compare themselves to others and want to "beat the competition" lack intrinsic motivation. It's exhausting and not sustainable, so avoid it by focusing on your own process, performance goals, and small wins.

Last, position yourself as an explorer and work on figuring out and tweaking the process to make it highly individualized to your own unique life and personal preferences. No two fitness journeys are the same. In Brad Stulberg's words, "Don't worry about being the best. Worry about being the best at getting better."[8]

PART II

NUTRITION

CHAPTER 5

Nutrition Fundamentals

Nutrition is a key building block to support our fitness goals and is the place where most of us get tripped up, which is not surprising, given the amount of confusing, conflicting, and complex information being circulated in the fitness industry. Credible fitness experts and even doctors preach the latest diets that are "proven" to induce weight loss. Yet these professionals contradict each other; no wonder we have a hard time figuring out who to believe.

Myths surrounding fitness and nutrition are perceived as truths by so many and have unfortunately become dogma, even though they've been disproven. We examine a few common myths later in this chapter.

Diet culture and the perceived need to fit a specific mold, as outlined by social media and companies in the business of weight loss, have become toxic. They have a pervasive effect on our society, and the spread of unhealthy advice has sadly led to eating disorder behavior, depression, and body-image issues among many of us. While the deleterious effects of diet culture are most prevalent with women, all genders are affected.

I have found a healthy way to approach nutrition. Although it can be easy to slip into eating disorder behavior, as I did and still struggle with from time to time, we can have a better relationship with food by doing some internal work and using the right framing. If we want to make changes to our bodies or even our minds, proper nutrition is so important. I want to stress that deprivation is not part of the equation here.

Find Your Stride's main message is that there is no one-size-fits-all diet or nutrition plan. We all have unique chemical makeups, genetics, and preferences, and so we should have a nutrition plan individually tailored to each and every one of us. Varying macronutrient splits (low carb/high fat or high carb/low fat) should be determined on an individual basis—not taken from the social media feed of an influencer who swears by flat-tummy teas and promotes waist cinchers.

As I lay out in the beginning of the book, the best way to approach nutrition is with the mindset of a scientist or explorer: Stay open-minded, absorb the information, and then experiment with different foods and macronutrient splits to figure out what works best for *you*. Keeping a food journal can help you strengthen your relationship with food. A journal is not just about meticulously tracking every calorie and macro that enters your body but about recording how different variations to your diet make you *feel*—how they affect your moods, energy levels, and satiety. No plan should leave you feeling depleted, low on energy, deprived, and moody. The correct plan should help you feel happy, healthy, energized, and satisfied. Figuring this out requires some experimentation and self-exploration, but it can be a rewarding and fun process.

In this part of the book, I lay out some important nutrition fundamentals, define some terminology to provide clarity surrounding confusing issues, provide a step-by-step process for determining your maintenance calories, and help you with an individualized macro split tailored to your body. I explain various approaches to nutrition that can support your individualized fitness goals (e.g., gaining muscle, losing body fat) and how you can leverage various nutrition timing strategies to capitalize on increased energy and performance in your training. Finally, we go over food tracking, eating behaviors, and supplements, and I showcase a few examples of meal plans you'll actually enjoy.

Quick disclaimer: While I do think counting calories and macros can help us become aware of our food choices, I also strongly believe that it's important to intertwine the principles of the intuitive eating approach developed by nutritionists Elyse Resch and Evelyn Tribole. Their approach is based on inner hunger signals as a guide to when and how much you should eat. I get into more details on intuitive eating later in this section. I realize these are conflicting schools of thought, but as noted initially, I'm a big proponent of mashing different strategies together, so I think there is something to learn from both.

Last, I want to mention that science is constantly changing and evolving as researchers continue to make new discoveries. New studies disproving long-held truths are published regularly. It's important to understand that this material presented here may have changed by the time you pick up this book. Therefore, I encourage you to scrutinize the information I give, use what you want, and remember to use this book as a guide, not gospel.

NUTRITION ESSENTIALS

The Basics of Energy Expenditure

In the simplest terms, the principle behind weight loss or weight gain stems from the law of thermodynamics. This is a law in physics surrounding the preservation of energy when added to a system. When applied to humans, we measure the energy component in the form of calories (a unit of energy). The law states that when energy is added to a system, we either expend that energy or store it.[1] For example, 1 kilocalorie is the amount of energy needed to raise the temperature of 1 kilogram of water by 1°C. Physiologically, if we consume more calories than we expend, we store the surplus as body fat.

The term *calorie* has a long history; while the origins aren't entirely clear, the original term *calorimeter* was coined by French chemist Antoine Lavoisier sometime between the years 1787 and 1824 and referred to a device that Lavoisier used to measure the production of heat.[2]

In 1863, *calorie* entered the English language from Adolphe Ganot's physics text, which defined a calorie as "the heat needed to raise the temperature of 1 kg of water from 0 to 1°C."[3] The calorie as used on food labels was popularized by an article published in 1887 by American chemist Wilbur Olin Atwater, titled "The Potential Energy of Food."[4]

Atwater burned each macronutrient (carbohydrate, protein, fat) in a calorimeter to devise a system that assigned the following values to the macronutrients: 4 kcal/g of protein, 4 kcal/g of carbohydrate, and 9 kcal/g of fat. An interesting article from the University of McGill compared the caloric content of a doughnut to that of a stick of dynamite (both have 450 kcal on average). The main difference? "The dynamite is released instantly when ignited, while the doughnut releases its energy content in the body more slowly. So you don't blow up from a doughnut. Not literally anyway."[5] Atwater's methods are still being used to evaluate the energy value of individual food items today.[6]

For our purposes, you can think of a calorie as synonymous with energy, and the theory behind "calories in versus calories out" is called energy balance. The famous mantra in the fitness industry states that to gain weight, you must be in a caloric surplus, and to lose weight, you must be in a caloric deficit. When the number of calories we consume outweighs the amount we burn, we're in a caloric surplus. When the number of calories we burn outweighs the amount we consume, we're in a caloric deficit. These are the bare-bones fundamentals of fluctuations in weight.

While there is some merit to the idea that being in caloric deficit makes you lose weight, there are also flaws with it. Many other factors are at play when trying to lose weight besides "being in a caloric deficit." Numerous studies have emerged that claim that caloric restriction may not be enough to induce weight loss over the long term. Drastically cutting calories and restricting food intake have been proven to reduce metabolic rates. A 2017 study by David Benton and Hayley Young states that "in the short term a reduction in energy intake is counteracted by mechanisms that reduce metabolic rate and increase calorie intake, ensuring the regaining of lost weight."[7] This, my friends, is what yo-yo dieting is all about.

Further, it is also entirely possible to lose weight when in a caloric surplus and gain weight while in a caloric deficit. We can lose or gain weight depending on variables that include loss or gain of muscle mass, water retention, bloating, and menstrual cycle (ladies, you know what I'm talking about). Certain supplements, such as creatine, can also influence your weight by causing water buildup in the muscles.

But for simplicity's sake, calories do matter. In fact, they are the most important determinant in a fat-loss plan. Generally speaking, if you eat in a surplus for prolonged periods, you will gain fat, and if you eat in a deficit long enough, you'll lose fat (and maybe muscle too, if you're cutting calories too aggressively and/or not getting adequate protein).

Next, let's define some key terms so we're all on the same page. I wish I had known these definitions at the start of my fitness journey, which would have prevented a lot of frustration and self-deprecating thoughts. But hey, live and learn.

Important Definitions

Many folks make the dire mistake of thinking that weight loss is synonymous with fat loss. It isn't. Let's differentiate the two for clarity's sake.

Weight is a person's body mass, or how heavy they are—it's most commonly measured in kilograms or pounds. Our weight can be affected by increases and decreases in body water, fat, and muscle. The scale is the most common and obvious way to measure an individual's weight.

Fat mass is the proportion of fat on our bodies. It can be measured by several different methods, including a caliper, a bio impedance (electronic scale), and the good old-fashioned analog method of a measuring tape. However, fat mass is most commonly taken as a percentage of overall body mass, referred to as *body fat percentage.*

Fat-free mass (FFM), also referred to as *lean body mass* (LBM), is calculated by taking the total body mass less the fat mass. Fat-free mass is what we want to try and grow or maintain.

Body recomposition is defined as losing body fat while concomitantly gaining lean muscle mass. In other words, body recomposition, or "body recomp," is what we're doing when we build muscle and lose body fat.

When most people set their physique goals, they're hoping to achieve one or more of the following: lose body fat, gain muscle, or preserve muscle mass. However, most people still say, "I want to lose weight." No, you want to lose body fat. Unless you are severely overweight or obese, weight change isn't as significant as other metrics. This distinction is important especially for those who are using the scale as the primary (or only) tracking device to determine their progress.

The scale never tells the whole story, and weight can fluctuate quite a bit from changes in both muscle mass and body water—both variables that are independent from fat loss or gain. You may, for example, see the scale number go down week over week and think you're making great progress, but in actuality, you may be losing muscle mass or just water. As discussed later in this chapter, the scale is not a tracking device I recommend using when trying to achieve body recomposition. It's fine if you use it in conjunction with other methods, but fair warning: the scale can be a deceiving liar that can make you feel discouraged and even give up your fitness goals altogether.

Further, using "weight" as an indicator of "health" is another misleading and problematic concern. Weight has historically been closely tied to BMI or body mass index—an outdated and inaccurate tool used to measure "health of an individual" by categorizing them as either a normal, healthy weight, underweight, overweight, or obese—a pretty black and white way of pigeon-holing someone into a box. To calculate BMI, the body mass (weight) of a person is divided by their height. The scale was adopted and popularized by the World Health Organization and is used almost dogmatically in the US health-care system. Sabrina Strings, in her fantastic book *Fearing the Black Body*, points out that many researchers and scholars agree that "[there] is racial bias in the BMI classification system."[8] Strings outlines a 2002 study that concludes, "[While] rates of obesity were shown to have been mounting nationwide, black women were singled out as having significant increases in their rates of [extreme obesity]."[9] Some studies have shown that black individuals have a lower body fat and higher lean muscle than white individuals, but at the same BMI, and therefore have less of a chance of developing disease related to obesity.[10]

A 2012 study titled "Ethnic-Specific BMI and Waist Circumference Thresholds" purported that black women can weigh significantly more than white women and still be considered healthy.[11] Another study showed that black women lose less weight than white women on the exact same calorie-restricted diet plan while keeping exercise the same.[12] BMI has long been debated, but it's mostly criticized for its oversimplification of diagnosing someone's weight, resulting in misdiagnosis in medicinal practice. Carly Stern, in the *Washington Post*, writes, "[Assumptions], practices and policies based on BMI adversely affect Americans of color by shaping the diagnoses they receive, treatment they access and stigma they may face."[13] I conclude by stating that we should move away from just looking at weight and what the scale spits out as it can indeed be problematic on an individual and societal level—especially toward black women.

Most diet plans preach that they will help you lose weight quickly, and to some extent, they may. But not necessarily the weight you want. The ketogenic diet, for instance, which severely restricts carbohydrate intake, forces the body into *ketosis*, which causes changes in body mass from water loss because carbohydrates cause the body to store extra water. You may also lose weight rapidly, but at the cost of your muscle mass. Again, not the changes you really want to make.

The takeaway here is to structure your nutrition plan to help you gain muscle and lose body fat (achieve body recomposition). You're going to want to make sure you're getting the nutrients required—and enough of them—to support your muscle growth and fat loss while also integrating a good resistance training program, which I cover in depth in Part III.

COMMON MYTHS

As stated before, fitness myths are pervasive in our society. Let's review two of these common myths, as they both relate to the topic of achieving body recomposition—losing fat and building muscle at the same time.

Myth 1: It's Not Possible to Gain Muscle in a Caloric Deficit

A popular misconception is that it's nearly impossible to lose body fat while simultaneously gaining muscle, or in other words, it's impossible to gain muscle while in a caloric deficit. This simply isn't true. The fact is, our internal systems for how the body distributes calories in the form of fat and muscle are separate. Therefore, it is quite possible to build muscle while in a caloric deficit—as long as we have adequate protein and a progressive resistance training plan in place.

But what does the science say? An article in the *Strength and Conditioning Journal* provides a meta-analysis that proves it is indeed possible to gain lean mass while simultaneously losing body fat.[14] There are some stipulations, of course. For example, you need to make sure you're getting adequate protein. In addition, research has shown that other variables affect our body recomposition efforts, including sleep, stress hormones, and metabolic rate, but these factors have been a bit tricky to measure and require further investigation. One more important factor to note is that it is indeed easier and typically faster to build muscle while eating in a caloric surplus, but this will likely result in some body fat coming along for the ride.

Myth 2: Only Novice Trainees or the Overweight Population Can Gain Muscle in a Caloric Deficit

Another popular myth is that only novice/beginner trainees or people who are overweight can capitalize on losing fat and building muscle simultaneously. While it may be easier for these folks to build muscle in a deficit, more experienced or resistance-trained individuals have these capabilities as well.

An abundance of scientific literature refutes this myth, including studies of elite gymnasts, rugby players, and other highly trained athletes. These groups were put on a diet of moderate caloric deficit, and guess what? They decreased fat mass while concurrently gaining lean body mass, although some of these studies showed only slight increases in lean body mass (especially in athletes with very low body fat percentages to begin with).

For example, one study put elite gymnasts on the ketogenic/carb-restricted diet in which they were allowed just under 2,000 calories a day while continuing to train as superhumans do. At the end of the study, they showed a decrease in body weight and fat mass and a slight, "non-significant" increase in muscle mass.[15]

Another study put 23 athletes on a calorie-restricted diet, adjusting their calories to aim to lose 0.5 kg of body weight per week, while also having them complete four resistance training sessions per week. The results showed a reduction in fat mass and an increase in lean body mass. Researchers concluded that to preserve and build lean body mass, you should aim for a body weight loss of 0.7% per week (or what is considered a moderate deficit—nothing too drastic).[16] I dive in to how to determine a moderate caloric deficit in the following chapters, so don't worry if you're feeling lost right now.

Personal trainer and fitness expert Menno Henselmans summarizes the research findings nicely, writing:

> [As] long as your body has sufficient stimulus to build muscle mass, which it has if your training program is optimized, it has both the means and the will to build muscle mass while simultaneously losing fat. There you go, muscle growth during a cut.[17]

NUTRITION FUNDAMENTALS TAKEAWAYS

Here are the key takeaways to understand as we move through the remainder of the book:

- Keep in mind the differences between weight loss and fat loss when setting your *aesthetic* fitness goals.

- The scale doesn't tell the whole story—you can be gaining weight and losing fat or the reverse, losing weight and gaining fat. So be wary of the scale.

- Body recomposition is losing body fat and gaining muscle simultaneously.

- It's possible for both sedentary and trained individuals to achieve body recomposition—losing body fat and gaining lean mass concurrently—while eating in a caloric deficit.

- It's also possible to gain weight, or more accurately, fat mass, while eating in a caloric deficit.

- It's easier for people with high body fat percentages, or those eating in a caloric surplus, to gain lean muscle mass with an adequate resistance training program. However, eating in a large caloric surplus also can add body fat, which is discussed in more detail in a later chapter.

CHAPTER 6

Determining Your Maintenance Calories

Now that I've covered some nutrition fundamentals and cleared up some definitions and common myths, let's get into the good stuff. I'll present a step-by-step process to help you figure out what and how much you should be eating to achieve your fitness goals. To preface what's to follow, this material involves some math. (Don't worry, it's simple math. I don't throw calculus equations at you or ask you to find the limit as z approaches a. If I can do it, you can do it too!)

Similar to changing an undesired behavior or habit, you need to have some level of awareness of your *energy balance*, which is how many calories you consume and burn in a given day to stay where you're at.

"Why would I want to know this?" you may ask. Well, to adjust our calories (up or down), we need a starting point—an equilibrium. Grasping this idea is essential because math is involved more than anything when it comes to changing our body composition. So, if you haven't done this exercise before, then it's time to pull out that calculator you haven't used since grade 12 math, dust it off, and go through these steps to determine how many calories you should eat to maintain your weight.

WHAT ARE MAINTENANCE CALORIES?

Maintenance calories are the exact number of calories to support your energy expenditure. To calculate this value, you need to calculate your total daily energy expenditure (TDEE). When most people think of TDEE, they think calories in (from eating) versus calories out (from exercise). However, we need to understand many more critical variables as well. So how do you determine your TDEE? By a very confusing and overwhelming formula:

$$TDEE = BMR + TEF + NEAT + PA$$

Umm, okay? Thanks, Em, you're making this crystal clear. So let's break this scientific jumble down to layman's terms.

BRM: This is your base metabolic rate, which is defined as the number of calories your body needs to perform its basic bodily functions: breathing, blood pumping through our veins, cell growth, and other processes we need to survive and thrive. Here's a fun fact: roughly 70% of the calories we burn in a given day are from doing absolutely nothing.

TEF: Did you know that different types of food have differing effects on your metabolic rate? You may have heard that spicy food, for instance, can increase your metabolism. TEF stands for the thermic effect of food, or the increase in our metabolic rate by the consumption, digestion, metabolism, and storage of food. Basically, our bodies expend energy (and burn calories) from the food we eat. Some types of food require more energy expenditure than others. Protein, for instance, has a higher thermic effect than both fat and carbs. So you'll likely burn more calories from eating eggs than a piece of toast.

NEAT: In addition to physical exercise, we also burn calories from other daily activities like talking with our hands, walking to our car, driving, cooking, cleaning, and so on. This part of the equation is called NEAT, or in confusing scientific terms, nonexercise activity thermogenesis.

PA: PA stands for physical activity, and this is intentionally planned exercise like running, swimming, and lifting. So no surprise here.

THE CALORIES WE BURN
IN EACH OF THE INPUTS

Did you know that most of the calories we burn during a given day are from the BRM part of the equation? About 60–70% of the calories we expend are from the physiological work our body performs. I would have guessed it was from movement, but no. Just by sitting, you burn a bunch of calories, which is why, before you even consider including exercise, you have a bulk of calories to play with in a given day. The TEF component obviously varies depending on the type of food we consume. Still, an average range lies in 6–12% of the total.[1] NEAT and PA make up the remainder of the equation and are also dependent on how active you are.

So now that you know the definitions, how many calories do you burn on average in a given day in each of the inputs, and how do you figure out this equation? How do you determine the thermal effect of food? Using a Fitbit, how can you measure the calories burned from breathing air?

You're probably thinking, *This is too much, Emily. I'm out.*

When I was going through this process, I felt the same way. Luckily, there are TDEE calculators. But, unluckily, these calculators offer a wide discrepancy of results. Most of these calculators ask for the following inputs: gender, age, weight, height, activity level, and some even ask for a body fat percentage.

I'll use myself as an example: I'm 139 lbs./63 kg, 5 ft. 6 in., and 32 years old; I will choose "heavy exercise (6–7 days per week)"; and my body fat is 13%. So here's what the differing calculators say:

Mayo Clinic calculator = 2,050 calories/day

MyFitnessPal = 2,150 calories/day

TDEEcalculator.net = 2,682 calories/day

That's a 632-calorie difference between the lower and higher ends!

So, what to do? Fitness tracking apps and TDEE calculators can be overly generous with the TDEE value and, on the reverse side, stingy when they spit out their recommended daily calorie expenditure. These calculators are also loaded with assumptions and don't reflect individualized factors such as your metabolism, genetics, the thermic effect of what you eat (TEF), and other considerations. Calorie calculators can be used as a guideline or starting point, but you need to do a bit of experimenting with them to really figure out what will work for you.

When I was first determining my caloric intake, I used the MyFitnessPal app as my baseline by adding in my stats listed previously and the amount of weight I wanted to lose per week, which ranged from 0.5 lbs. to 2 lbs. per week. This gave me a ballpark number of calories I got to play with in a given day. The consensus on the web is that most people use the TDEE calculator at https://tdeecalculator.net, but I personally found its calculation to be too high. If I ate that many calories in a day, I would definitely see my body fat go up, even with the considerable amount of cardio I do each day.

Since you made it this far in the book, you likely have your experimenter hat on, and I recommend not using the calculators. I suggest, instead, using the following two methods, which take more factors into account—even though these two methods also have some drawbacks:

1. The analog method of tracking everything you eat and your weight for at least one week

2. The Harris-Benedict equation, which calculates TDEE using your BMR and applying an activity multiplier

The first method is more work, but it's definitely the most accurate. The second method is quick, and I've found that it has been the most consistent of all other formulas but perhaps not as accurate as the analog method. Choose one method, or do both and compare them if you're a nerd like me.

The Analog Method of Calculating Maintenance Calories

Our weight fluctuates daily and so does our calorie intake. So the best way to figure out the correlation between how much we eat and how much we weigh is to track both every day for one to two weeks and then take the averages of each. Our bodies are dynamic and always changing, so there's never a sure bet. This analog method is pretty common in the world of bodybuilding and has been adopted by several coaches in the industry. Physique coach Paul

Revelia calls this method a "diet and activity recall."[2] Dr. Eric Helms also gets clients to put in some groundwork before he puts together a specific nutrition plan to align with their goals.[3] What follows are the action steps to take if you want to follow the analog method.

STEP 1: THE "INTAKE PERIOD"

For one to two weeks, track every single thing you put into your body using a calorie tracking app while also taking daily body weight measurements using a standard scale. You can keep track of all this data in a spreadsheet, a piece of paper, or the downloadable chart at https://www.emilyrudow.com/findyourstride/resources.

STEP 2: ANALYZE THE DATA

Once you've collected the data, you'll want to figure out the amount of weight you've gained, lost, or maintained by determining seven-day averages for each week. Then observe the correlation with your calorie intake.

STEP 3: APPLY A FORMULA COMPARING THE RELATIONSHIP BETWEEN THE TWO WEEKS

Note that 3,500 calories roughly equates to 1 lb. or 0.5 kg of body weight (lost or gained). Helms uses this knowledge as a rough estimation to determine the following:

- 500-calorie surplus/deficit per day is roughly 1 lb. or 0.5 kg gained/lost per week

- 1,000-calorie surplus/deficit per day is roughly 2 lbs. or 1 kg gained/lost per week

Look at the change in your average body weight in week 1 compared to week 2, and then you can see the relationship with your caloric intake and how it is affecting your body weight.

EXAMPLE

Step 1: The "Intake Period"

When I conducted this experiment, I used MyFitnessPal to track my caloric intake and a standard scale for my body weight. I added the total amount of calories I ate in a given day into a spreadsheet along with my weight. I weighed myself as soon as I woke up to provide some consistency. Say on Monday I ate 2,200 calories and weighed 140 lbs., I'd log my table as so:

Day	Calories	Weight
Monday	2,200	140

However, I think it's better if you input the calories you ate *the day before* and the current day's weight, so that the data better represents the impact the calories consumed the previous day had on today's weight. Instead of using today's calories, I would use Sunday's calories (2,500 calories) and Monday's weight on the same line:

Day	Calories	Weight
Monday	2,500	140

Now that we've got that detail out of the way, here's a step-by-step guide on how to calculate your maintenance calories:

1. Track calories and weight daily for two weeks.

2. Total up week 1 calories and weight and divide by seven.

3. Total up week 2 calories and weight and divide by seven.

Here's what my two-week period looked like:

Week 1

Date	Calories	Weight (lbs.)
April 1	1,900	141
April 2	1,807	140
April 3	1,977	139
April 4	2,418	139
April 5	2,005	137
April 6	2,268	137
April 7	2,000	138

Week 2

Date	Calories	Weight (lbs.)
April 8	3,000	139
April 9	1,970	141
April 10	1,930	138
April 11	2,045	137
April 12	2,000	137
April 13	2,400	139
April 14	1,850	139

I want you to notice a few things. First, look at how much my weight fluctuated each day (there were a few days where it stayed the same) and how wildly my caloric intake changed. This is important because (1) our bodies are dynamic and our energy needs differ each day, and (2) the scale changes all the time—*I told you*. We circle back to this later (just keep it in your back pocket for now).

Once I captured my data for both weeks, I totaled each week's weight and calories then divided both by seven. This gave me a daily calorie and weight average for each week. During this trial period, I tried to stay consistent with my workouts and didn't incorporate any longer runs or abnormal workouts.

Step 2: Analyze Results

Here were my results over the two-week period:

> Week 1: 138.71 lbs., average 2,054 calories/day
>
> Week 2: 138.57 lbs., average 2,171 calories/day

On average, I lost 0.14 lbs. (or 0.063 kg) on 2,171 calories.

Step 3: Apply a Formula to Figure Out Your Maintenance Calories

I next used the following formula I learned from Helms to determine my maintenance calories. First, you calculate your caloric deficit or surplus:

> 1,000 kcal (per day) × the amount of weight gained
> or lost (week 1 weight minus week 2 weight in
> *kilograms*) = caloric surplus/deficit

In practice, I take the 1,000 kcal and multiply it by the 0.63 kg (amount of weight lost):

> 1,000 kcal (per day) × 0.063 kg (the amount of weight
> lost/gained in kg) = 63 caloric deficit

Then, I take the caloric deficit (63 in this example) and add it to the number of calories (how much I lost/gained) to get my maintenance calories:

Maintenance = 2,171 calories + 63 = 2,234 calories/day

A note for women: Ladies, try to do this *after* your period, because hormones mess everything up. I have an insatiable appetite the week leading up to my period, I feel bloated, and my boobs feel like sandbags.

Just be aware that your maintenance calories will not remain constant, and neither will your weight (these variables fluctuate daily), but by doing the groundwork, it will provide you with a good baseline to manipulate the calorie inputs and outputs.

Calculating TDEE Using the Harris-Benedict Equation

Let me introduce you to the famous Harris-Benedict equation, a formula that was derived from a study by botanist and biometrician James Arthur Harris and chemist Francis Gano Benedict. First published in 1919, the Harris-Benedict equation is one of the oldest and most commonly used formulas for calculating TDEE. Since then, it's been modified to provide more accuracy by Mifflin and colleagues in 1990.[4] While there are a bunch of these formulas out there, the Harris-Benedict equation has provided the most consistent results over time. However, note that it's still a calculation and thus provides just a guesstimate. Here's the formula:

TDEE = BMR × Activity multiplier

Recall that your BMR is the number of calories you burn when your body is at rest. Once you have your BMR, you can use an activity multiplier based on how much activity you do in a given day (your work, exercise, and so on). And that's it. This method for calculating TDEE is much simpler than the analog method and only requires a few simple steps.

STEP 1: CALCULATE BMR

To calculate your BMR, you just need to know your weight and height. Oh, yeah, you also need to know your age, which I'm really hoping you do.

You can choose to do the calculations using the imperial system (used in the United States) or the metric system, and I've included both.

METRIC SYSTEM

Men BMR = [10 × weight (kg)] + [6.25 × height (cm)] − [5 × age (years)] + 5

Women BMR = [10 × weight (kg)] + [6.25 × height (cm)] − [5 × age (years)] − 161

IMPERIAL AND US SYSTEMS

Men BMR = 66.47 + (6.24 × weight in lbs.) + (12.7 × height in inches) − (6.755 × age in years)

Women BMR = 655.1 + (4.35 × weight in lbs.) + (4.7 × height in inches) − (4.7 × age in years)

As an example, this is how I would calculate my BMR using the imperial/US systems. I'm 5 ft. 6 in. (so 66 inches), I'm 32 years old, and I weigh 139 lbs.

Women BMR = 655.1 + (4.35 × 139 lbs.) + (4.7 × 66 inches) − (4.7 × 32 years)

BMR = 1,420

STEP 2: ACTIVITY MULTIPLIER

The final step in this method is to determine the average amount of activity you do in a given day and multiply the associated multiplier by your BMR.

Sedentary = 1.2 ×

If you don't exercise much, work a desk job, have long commutes to and from work, or your body is simply at rest most of the day, then you can use the sedentary classification.

Light activity = 1.375 ×

Say you work out one to three days per week at the gym or you play some sports, maybe go for daily walks, but still work a desk job, you can classify your activity as light.

Moderate activity = 1.55 ×

If you work out or play sports three to five days per week or incorporate some walking or other forms of activity (maybe cleaning, gardening, etc.) in your days, you can put yourself in the moderate activity level.

Very active = 1.725 ×

If you're an avid gym goer or play sports six to seven days per week, incorporate other movement/activity in your day, and are on your feet for work for most of the day, you can classify yourself as very active.

Very, very active = 1.9 ×

This is next-level activity. Only classify yourself here if you work out six to seven days per week and have a physically demanding job and/or are training two times per day in some cases (elite athletes may fit into this category).

As an example, since I work out seven days per week and also incorporate 30-minute walks five to six days per week, but also work a desk job, I would put myself in the *very active* category and give myself a classification of 1.725. I would then calculate my TDEE by multiplying my BMR by my activity multiplier.

TDEE = 1,420 (BMR) × 1.725 (activity multiplier)

Maintenance = 2,450 calories

As you can see, my BMR overshoots my calories by a bit from the analog method's calculations (about 216 calories over), but it's not bad!

FITNESS TRACKERS

Before we move on to calculating macros, I'd like to quickly discuss the use of fitness trackers. If on some days you exercise more than normal (for example, run a half marathon), your caloric needs will definitely increase. This is where having a rough estimate of the additional calories burned comes in handy. However, there doesn't seem to be any general consensus on the best way to get this estimate. So I share here what works best for me, and you can decide whether you want to adopt the same practice.

Fitness trackers are terrible at measuring our energy expenditure, so be wary. You know what fitness trackers are good for? They are best at measuring your steps and your heart rate *sometimes*, and some trackers are better than others.

A few fitness tracking apps will allow you to add the activity, duration of time, and weight that can give you a rough estimate of the calories you burned. My rule of thumb is to enter in the calories burned from cardio only (running, cycling, or walking) because resistance training is too difficult to measure or guess. I use MyFitnessPal to log my daily exercise time, and I find that the calorie expenditure is pretty consistent with other calculators. When I log my exercise time, for instance, I'll choose "activity > run" and then pick my pace (or close to it) and add the duration. The app will then automatically add the calories burned from exercise to my TDEE. I recommend using a calculator or app rather than what your fitness tracker spits out. Even if the tracker claims that it's accurate, it isn't. Too many studies have demonstrated how far off the calorie estimate is on fitness trackers.[5] Because of their unreliability, I recommend using fitness trackers to measure your activity metrics (pace, duration, steps, etc.), but that's about it.

CHAPTER 7

Macronutrients and Micronutrients

Now that you have an understanding of your caloric needs, it's time to move on to discuss macronutrients and how to calculate the ideal macro split to help you achieve your goals. But first, let's start with the basics.

WHAT ARE MACROS?

Macros are the nutrients our body needs in larger quantities to provide us with sustained energy. Consisting of carbohydrates, fats, and proteins, each macro plays a unique role in our body's ability to operate efficiently. The premise of counting macros is founded on the basis that not all calorie forms are created equal, which is true. Measured in grams, macros can be split in various ways depending on your nutritional needs and fitness goals. For instance, an average macro split for a normal person might be high carb/moderate protein/moderate fat (45–65% carbs/10–35% protein/20–35% fat). Whereas, a low carb/moderate fat/moderate protein split might be broken down like this: 15–25% carbs/40–50% protein/30–35% fat.

Counting macros can also be called flexible eating, which is giving people permission to eat what they want, as long as it fits into their macros (more on this later). However, that doesn't necessarily mean you *should* eat anything and everything you want within your macro count. Incorporating healthy, nutrient-rich foods into your diet will provide your body with energy, good cognitive performance, and optimal bodily functioning, which you probably already know. There are some best practices that can help you have a healthy relationship with each macronutrient and support your body recomposition goals.

And that's just the thing: not all of our bodies operate on the same playing field. There have been numerous examples of people achieving their "ideal body" in more unconventional ways. Michael Matthew's best seller, *Bigger Leaner Stronger*, profiles a professor who lost 27 pounds on a diet consisting of Twinkies, protein shakes, Doritos, Oreos, and other sugary snacks featuring my main gal, Little Debbie. This example might be a bit more of an anomaly, but the point I'm trying to make is that it's important to incorporate a progressive training plan and also ensure that you're getting adequate protein.

THE IDEAL MACRO SPLIT

John Romaniello, on his blog *Roman Fitness Systems*, has a great analogy comparing nutrition with baking. John writes, "Not only do you need the exact right ingredients, you need the exact amounts of them. And you have to add them in precisely the right order. If you mess up one single piece of that, everything pretty much collapses."[1]

I wouldn't necessarily say that your nutrition plan would "collapse" if you don't follow an exact split, but some awareness of your macronutrient consumption is needed to help support your training and fitness goals. You do need to put the correct ingredients (macro- and micronutrients) into your body. Therefore, it's important to understand what each of the macronutrients are, what role they play, and how you can use each one to propel you down the right path to support your goals.

However—spoiler alert—there isn't an exemplary macronutrient split to follow. I get into the carbs versus fats debate shortly, but when it comes to counting macros, the most important one to pay attention to is your protein intake. You should focus on your protein intake first, and then split out your carbs and fats from there.

While some of the following material is not the most exciting (there's no easy way to spice this stuff up), I think it's important to present scientific literature in a matter-of-fact way, showing both sides, any existing controversies, and noting when more investigation is needed to reach a conclusion. So let's dive in!

PROTEIN

If you're going to skim over anything in this book, please don't skim over this section. Get your highlighter, calculator, and sticky notes out! Protein is the most important macronutrient to cover because it provides the building blocks to any muscle building or fat-loss plan. Which is why, of course, we should pay attention to figuring out how much protein we *really* need.

What Is Protein?

From a molecular standpoint, the protein molecule is comprised of long-chain amino acids and plays various roles in our bodies. Protein molecules repair and build muscle tissue, improve our immune systems, fight infection,[2] balance pH levels,[3] transport nutrients to different parts of our bodies,[4] and have beneficial effects on our metabolisms.[5] Proteins are found in a wide array of animal and plant-based foods but have the highest concentration in animal products and by-products (meat, dairy, etc.).

High-Protein Diet for Body Recomposition

Decades of scientific research have suggested that a high-protein diet can help us build muscle, preserve lean muscle mass, and accelerate fat loss. Specifically, the amino acid leucine that is found in protein can play an important role in inducing muscle protein synthesis (MPS). MPS is a process that occurs when our body uses protein to help repair damaged muscle tissue after exercise. Following are a few reasons why protein can aid in your fitness and health efforts.

Increased satiety: High-protein diets have been proven to increase satiety levels (compared to carbs and fats) with the same caloric intake, which can help us lower our energy intake and thus better promote our fat-loss efforts.[6]

Thermic effect: Protein intake is associated with an increase in thermogenesis. Protein has about double the thermic effect of carbs and fats, meaning that your body can burn about twice the number of calories digesting and absorbing protein as it does with carbs or fats.[7]

Growth and maintenance of fat-free mass: Some studies show a high protein intake can have a "stimulatory effect on muscle protein anabolism," which can help us build and retain lean muscle mass while boosting our metabolism.[8]

Determining Your Protein Targets

How much protein do you really need? Well, like anything fitness related, it depends on many factors: your current weight, body fat percentage, body recomposition goals, genetics, preexisting kidney disease or issues, whether you eat a calorie surplus or deficit, and a laundry list of other factors. Having so many variables to consider and contradictory opinions on protein consumption in academia, pop culture, and social media understandably causes much confusion.

Scientists have published differing protein target ranges from 0.7 g/lb. (1.6 g/kg) of body weight all the way up to 1.4 g/lb. (3.1 g/kg). I present you with a few different models and studies and then provide the recommendation I've landed on based on cross-referencing multiple sources and verifying the range with experts in the field.

THE LOW END OF PROTEIN INTAKE (0.7 G/LB. OR 1.6 G/KG)

A popular and widely known meta-analysis concluded that protein intakes greater than about 0.73 g/lb. (1.62 g/kg) *do not* contribute to gains in fat-free mass.[9] In other words, any intake over that amount does not support the growth of any additional lean muscle mass. The researchers reviewed 49 protein intake studies with close to 2,000 participants, which sounds legit, right? One important caveat: The majority of the study's participants were untrained individuals (that is, they didn't participate in a regular resistance training regimen) who were not eating in a caloric deficit or trying to lose body fat. If you're a resistance-trained athlete integrating a progressive training plan and *especially* in a caloric deficit, this suggestion is probably too low for you.

THE 1 G/LB. OR 2.2 G/KG OF BODY WEIGHT RULE
FOR DETERMINING PROTEIN INTAKE

Generally speaking, the 1 g/lb. of body weight rule of thumb has become common among physique coaches and can provide a good guideline for individuals within an average weight range. However, in fitness YouTuber Jeff Nippard's video "The Science behind My Protein Diet," he points out that extremes in weight are a major flaw in this ratio. For example, Nippard mentioned that a 300 lb. person would be advised to ingest 300 g of protein on a given day, which is indeed overkill.[10] Nippard also mentions that this rule is a pretty good standard, as it tends to overestimate protein intake, the math can't get any simpler, and it's quite easy to remember. When it comes to fitness, sometimes the simplest way can steer you on the right path.

THE MEDIAN RANGE OF PROTEIN INTAKE
(0.7 G/LB.–1.1 G/LB. OR 1.6 G/KG–2.4 G/KG)

Now we're starting to inch closer to a reasonable range. Rather than examining untrained individuals, a 2018 study looked at elite athletes—highly trained individuals with typically lower body fat percentages. The study concluded that "high-quality weight loss" is important to elites to "maintain their muscle (engine) and shed unwanted fat mass, potentially improving athletic performance."[11] The researchers recommend a protein range of 1.6 g/kg to 2.4 g/kg, which depends on a few factors: the "severity" of the caloric deficit and the intensity level and type of training you're doing. If you're eating in a caloric deficit or are already very lean (low body fat percentage), they advise moving to the higher end of the protein range.[12]

THE EXPERT RANGE OF PROTEIN INTAKE

The consensus among some of the top fitness experts in the field (Dr. Eric Helms and Menno Henselmans, among others) is to aim for at least 0.91 g/lb. (2 g/kg) of body weight or more of protein per day. The range that Helms and Henselmans, among other experts, agree on is 0.82 g/lb. to 1.23 g/lb. (1.8 g/kg to 2.7 g/kg), with 0.82 g/lb. (1.8 g/kg) being the lowest intake you should aim for. Henselmans explains that within that range, you generally won't experience any major or even noticeable differences in performance or body composition.[13] People who have a progressive training plan, are eating in a caloric deficit, and trying to lose body fat should go higher on the protein intake range.

When calculating protein targets, it's best to calculate a range. Take the lower end of your range and multiply it by your body weight (in kilograms). Then take your upper range and multiply your body weight (in kilograms), and—voilà!—you have your range.

I typically aim for between about 1 g/lb. (2.3 g/kg) and 1.1 g/lb. (2.5 g/kg) of protein per day, but if I go over, then it's an added bonus! Here's what my calculations look like:

$$63 \text{ kg (139 lbs.)} \times 2.3 \text{ g protein} = {\sim}145 \text{ g/day}$$
$$63 \text{ kg (139 lbs.)} \times 2.5 \text{ g protein} = {\sim}158 \text{ g/day}$$

My daily protein range is 145–158 g/day.

Take a minute to pause, pull out that calculator, and use the above equation on yourself. I want to once again emphasize how important it is to hit your protein targets. Start by calculating your goal, write it out, and even post it on your fridge!

Is Too Much Protein Bad for You?

Before we conclude this macronutrient, it's worth mentioning yet another point of contention about protein intake: Can too much protein have deleterious effects on your kidneys and bones? Let's dive in to each of these points and see what the current discourse suggests.

BAD FOR YOUR KIDNEYS?

"Too much protein is bad for your kidneys" is one phrase I've heard way too many times and that I've also fallen prey to. Where did this idea come from? Well, an old hypothesis was the idea that protein put added stress on the kidneys to remove waste (a process called hyperfiltration).[14] There is a bit of truth to this statement; however, any negative side effects of a high-protein diet can be linked to people with preexisting kidney issues or diseases.[15] Several studies conducted on healthy adults or those with normal kidney function have shown that high-protein diets *do not* aversely influence our kidneys at all.

BAD FOR YOUR BONES?

Another common myth is that too much protein can be bad for your bones. The theory states that since protein can increase acid in the body, our bodies will extract calcium out of our bones and use it to neutralize the acid, which may potentially lead to osteoporosis. While some studies have shown this to be the case in the short term, there are no long-term studies that show any negative effects on bone health from protein intake.[16] One 2017 meta-analysis looked at 16 randomized control trials and 20 prospective cohort studies on high-protein intake evaluating the effects high-protein diets had on bone health. The study concluded that higher protein intake has absolutely no adverse effects. In fact, evidence was uncovered to support "positive trends" on bone mineral density.[17]

A final study showed that a high-protein diet combined with a heavy resistance training program resulted in a greater decrease in fat mass and body fat percentage in trained men and women, which we knew already. But the study also concludes that "there is no evidence that consuming a high-protein diet has any harmful effects."[18]

Takeaways

If you're looking to make body recomposition changes, protein is the most important macronutrient to focus on. While there are differing schools of thought on how much protein you should consume daily, the expert consensus is that we should aim for at least 2 grams of protein per kilogram of body weight. If you're eating in a caloric deficit, it's better to go higher. Unless you have preexisting kidney issues, there is no scientific evidence to suggest that eating a high-protein diet is bad for your kidneys or for your bones. Protein is an essential building block for muscle growth. With the combination of the thermic effect and protein's satiating ability, protein is a strong ally in helping you build muscle and lose body fat.

CARBOHYDRATES

Carbohydrates are like reality TV—people tend to demonize them and deny that they exist in their life. However, we all have a fondness for them—even if we're embarrassed to admit it. The most notorious carbs (I'm talking sugars, desserts, breads, etc.) are definitely enjoyable in the moment, but some of us experience the post-carb consumption slump shortly thereafter. We love eating them but unwittingly feel a ping of guilt afterward because of carbs' reputation as one of the biggest catalysts for weight gain. No other macronutrient is a bigger point of contention than carbs. It's important, therefore, to take you through what a carbohydrate actually is and present the latest research on the impact carbohydrates can have on your fat-loss efforts. My hope is that you'll stop demonizing them, which I certainly did early on in my weight-loss journey. Realize that carbs are more complex than most people know (pun intended). Just open your mind and heart to our dear little carbie. You may even come to revere this so-called enemy.

What Are Carbohydrates?

From a purely nondescript, scientific standpoint, carbohydrates are defined as a combination of carbon, hydrogen, and oxygen (in the ratio of 1:2:1). Dietary carbs can be either digested or transformed into glucose, which can then be used by our bodies as a source of energy.[19]

The carbohydrate food categories include fruits, sugars (processed and unprocessed), vegetables, fibers, and legumes. Each carbohydrate can be broken down further by a molecular structure, which I rudimentarily define (to not confuse you with a bunch of scientific jargon) as follows.

- *Monosaccharide:* simple sugars that are the "building blocks" of a carb. Examples include glucose, fructose (honey, fruits).[20]

- *Disaccharide:* compound containing two monosaccharides. Table sugar, for example, contains a molecule of fructose and a molecule of glucose ("double sugar"). Other examples include maltose and lactose.

- *Oligosaccharide:* contains three to six monosaccharide units that aren't frequently found in natural sources but are produced by breaking down complex carbohydrates (polysaccharides).[21]

- *Polysaccharides:* long chains of monosaccharides that vary in size and complexity. Examples include cellulose and starches (bread, potatoes).[22]

Are you lost yet? Me too. Let's move on to your second helping of scientific jargon.

Carbs can then be broken out even further by their type, structure, and other factors.

SIMPLE CARBS

These are simple short-chain compounds containing monosaccharides or disaccharides and can be used by our body quickly as a source of energy. Consuming simple carbs causes a fast rise in both blood sugar and insulin secretion. The rapid rise in blood sugar can give us a quick high, followed by a precipitous crash, which can leave us moody, tired, and hungry (usually for more simple carbs). Some examples include chocolate, desserts, honey, white sugar, and just about everything else that is delicious.

COMPLEX CARBS

Complex carbs contain three or more sugars (oligosaccharides or polysaccharides) bonded together in a more complex chemical structure. These carbs take a lot longer to digest than simple carbs and have a slower release of energy and increase in blood sugar. Examples include legumes, apples, oatmeal, quinoa, and sweet potatoes.

In short, the main difference between simple and complex carbs can be defined by the chemical structure and how quickly the body digests and absorbs each one.

STARCHES

To further confuse you, complex carbs can be broken out even further into different types of starches. These contain large amounts of the molecule glucose and, physiologically speaking, provide us with the energy to support brain function.[23] Potatoes, wheat products, and pasta are all classified as starches.

FIBER

Plant-based foods contain dietary fiber that cannot be digested by the body. But as fiber passes through the digestive tract, it provides a myriad of health-related benefits aside from nutrition. Fiber is broken out into two distinct types: soluble and insoluble. The main difference is that soluble fiber dissolves in water, whereas insoluble fiber doesn't. Most fiber-rich foods contain both types of fiber, with a heavier skew toward insoluble.[24]

Insoluble fiber absorbs water in the intestines and softens the stool. It aids the digestive track and helps provide predictable and smooth-sailing bowel movements. Insoluble fiber can also help reduce the risk of diabetes. Examples of insoluble fiber include seeds, potato skins, nuts, and wheat bran.

After soluble fiber dissolves in water, it ferments in the large intestine where it produces the hormones peptide (GLP-1) and peptide YY (PYY), which both help with satiety.[25] Soluble fiber also assists in stabilizing blood sugars and cholesterol. Some examples of soluble fiber include peas, barley, oats, and strawberries.

To summarize, eat your fiber, kiddies. It will help you poop and feel full.

The Glycemic Index

In the 1980s, Professor David Jenkins developed the glycemic index (GI) as a system for ranking carbohydrates based on their immediate effect on blood glucose after carb consumption. At first, the system was used to help people with diabetes make smart food choices and opt for foods with a lower GI. The ranking system is out of 100: low is less than 55, medium is 55–69, and high is 70 or greater.[26] Foods with low GI include green vegetables, beans, chickpeas, and oat bran. Medium-GI foods include bananas, whole wheat bread, brown rice, and pineapple. High-GI foods include white rice, white bread, and corn.

Following this system exclusively, however, presents some flaws. In Michael Matthew's book *Bigger Leaner Stronger*, he highlights a shortcoming of the GI system: a Snickers bar has a lower GI than oatmeal. It's also interesting to note that a green banana is ranked as medium-GI food, but when it ripens, it moves to the high-GI category. This change is due to the starches in the banana starting to break down into sugars as the banana ripens.

Foods with a lower GI can typically help with the overall health of the overweight/obese or diabetic populations. But if you're already healthy and aren't diabetic, GI might not matter all that much. Menno Henselmans concluded from a number of studies that GI doesn't have an effect on "healthy" individuals. Henselmans found that when it comes to strength training (anaerobic activity), the GI load doesn't influence performance in the gym whatsoever.[27]

What about the Low-Carb Diet?

The myth that "carbs make you fat" is probably the most timeworn statement in the fitness industry, and let me tell you, this myth hasn't aged well. A pioneer in the "low-carb diet" canon that I was equally amused and horrified to discover was a book by Robert Cameron called *The Drinking Man's Diet*. Published in 1964, the book became so popular that it went on to sell 2.4 million copies. This fad diet was a high-fat, high-protein regimen with—you guessed it—copious amounts of alcohol. Cameron claimed that to lose weight, you just needed to eat less than 60 g of carbohydrates per day and could eat as much fat as you wanted, all while crushing as many spirits as your heart desired. However, this book didn't gain much traction in the scientific community (thankfully) and was harshly criticized. A 1965 piece in *Time* magazine gave a sharp but deserved criticism of Cameron's work, claiming that "the book's contents are a cocktail of wishful thinking, a jigger of nonsense and a dash of sound advice."[28] Ouch.

In the 1990s, Dr. Robert Atkins popularized the low-carb, high-fat diet with his book *The Diet Revolution*. Atkins claimed that a low-carb diet forced the body to use fat stores instead of glycogen (the body's go-to) as the primary energy source. This process is known as ketosis.[29] Atkins's claims were widely criticized for close to 30 years, and only recently did the ketogenic diet craze swing the pendulum once again in favor of the low-carb diet.

The Carbohydrate-Insulin Model

You've likely heard the many controversies surrounding the hormone insulin and its supposed effect on weight gain. The carbohydrate-insulin model (CIM), developed by David Ludwig and Cara Ebbeling, attempts to poke holes in the conventional model of obesity: the school of thought that posits that calories in versus calories out, or *energy balance*, is a key determinant in weight loss and weight gain. Ludwig and Ebbeling argue that the conventional model fails to provide a complete explanation for the obesity epidemic (aside from the supposed lack of willpower and self-control in the obese population). The main question posed by the CIM is the following: Is a calorie a calorie? In other words, are all calories treated equal when it comes to weight gain?

CIM's main arguments center around the types of food you eat rather than the quantity of food you're ingesting—specifically, how high-GI carbohydrates (e.g., refined sugars) affect blood insulin levels. The argument goes a little something like this: When we eat carbohydrates, our insulin spikes, causing our bodies to transport this fuel and deposit it into our fat cells (instead of sending that fuel to the rest of the body). The result? Ludwig and Ebbeling write, "Consequently, fewer calories remain available in the blood stream for use by the rest of the body, driving hunger and overeating."[30] This makes sense. We eat a bagel and drink some juice and are hungry within an hour. Foods that are high in refined carbs cause our blood sugars to spike and then drop dramatically, cueing hunger and causing us to eat more. In short, refined carbohydrates are not very satiating. It's worth noting that protein also induces insulin but at the same time produces a catabolic hormone that "antagonizes" it—having an almost neutralizing effect. Dietary fat has little direct impact on our insulin levels, which has formed a strong argument for the high-fat, low-carb diet. Sounds compelling.

However, here's where the CIM falls apart: insulin plays a larger role in our body than just storing fat.

Insulin moves glucose into your muscles and other vital organs and stimulates lipogenesis—a process in which fatty acids are transported from your blood into your fat cells.[31] Carbohydrates can be converted and stored as fat in the body, but only if you're in a caloric surplus. If your body doesn't have the excess energy, there won't be anything to store. In short, we can't blame insulin levels as the sole contributor behind the obesity epidemic.

Innumerable studies have disproved the hypothesis that a high-carbohydrate diet causes weight gain or makes you fat. A 2017 meta-analysis titled "Obesity Energetics: Body Weight Regulation and the Effects of Diet Composition" looked at 32 controlled feeding studies. The study concluded that there are no weight-loss benefits from eating a particularly low-carb or high-carb diet as long as energy balance is maintained and sufficient protein requirements are met.[32] When it comes down to it, energy balance (calories in versus calories out) is the fundamental determinant of weight loss or weight gain.

However, I would be remiss not to mention that low-carb diets have worked for many people and can be an effective strategy for weight loss in particular groups (for example, those with type 2 diabetes). There is also merit in the CIM in that a diet high in refined carbohydrates (processed carbs, refined sugars, and some starch categories) can lead to weight gain if eaten in excess. These types of carbohydrates are indeed less satiating and tend to keep you less full compared to other macronutrients, which can cause you to reach for the snack cupboard more frequently. If we eat a diet that's high carb, low protein, and low fat, then we'll likely put ourselves into a caloric surplus. Last, carbohydrate-rich foods can also lead to water retention in the body, which can give an illusion that you are "gaining weight" and can throw you off kilter if you're looking at the scale too often.[33]

How Carbs Can Support Our Training Goals

Incorporating complex carbohydrates that are high in fiber can aid our digestive track, keep us satiated, and provide us with the fastest source of energy. All these benefits can help support our daily bodily functioning and improve performance in training.

Unlike fats and proteins, carbohydrates are the only macro that doesn't have a minimum dietary requirement. While many populations flourish off a carb-rich diet, others thrive off a diet predominately high in fat with very little carb intake (for example, certain indigenous populations).[34] I think this is one of the reasons why there's so much confusion surrounding carbohydrates. We tend to oversimplify without knowing the exact quantities to include. *How much is too much?*

As with proteins, your carb intake will depend on the type of activity you're engaging in, as well as your gender, personal preferences, genetics, and carbohydrate tolerance. In short, it's contingent on *you*. Let's review each consideration.

TYPE OF ACTIVITY

For endurance and high-intensity sports like running and ice hockey, our glycogen stores deplete much quicker, than with, say, weight training. Carbs can provide prolonged forms of energy to fuel performance. The average weight lifter doesn't deplete as much glycogen when working out as a runner might and can squeak by with eating fewer carbs and supplementing pre-workout with more protein and/or fat. Some studies have shown that weight lifting results in only a 26–28% glycogen depletion.[35]

For high-intensity activity—sprinting, cycling, or endurance sports—glycogen stores decrease at a much more rapid rate and can benefit from a high-carb meal pre- and intra-workout, which provides the quickest release of energy to fuel performance. If you're doing lower-intensity exercise, such as steady-state cardio or light jogging, your body will likely use fat or protein for fuel instead of carbs (more on this later).

For my longer runs that are over 13 miles, I'll typically eat some oats mixed with protein powder and nut butter, giving my body a good mix of carbs, protein, and fat. For my daily 5-mile runs, I will opt for a lighter snack like a protein bar or some Greek yogurt, almonds, and half of a pear. I've experimented with my macro split quite a bit over the years, and I encourage you to do the same. However, a good rule of thumb is if you're planning on doing a high-intensity or long endurance workout, it's typically better to up the carbs.

GENDER

Recent scientific studies concluded that carb intakes affect men's and women's performance differently.[36] One study showed that women burn more lipid (fat) and fewer carbs than men during endurance exercise because of the role of the 17 beta-estradiol hormone (a major female sex hormone produced by the ovaries).[37] Further research studied endurance athletes and the effect that carbs had on glycogen concentration. The study concluded that after ingesting carbs, men saw an increase in muscle glycogen, whereas women didn't.[38] This means that women may benefit from eating more fats than carbs, and generally speaking, women don't need as many carbohydrates to fuel exercise as men do.

However, even though studies have shown carbs to be more beneficial to men than to women, I don't want you to just take this advice at face value. Some women perform better with a high-carb intake, and some men perform better with a low-carb intake. Once again, I encourage you to try it out for yourself. As a cis woman, I personally don't perform best physically or cognitively when I eat a high-fat diet, so carbs make up a large portion of my macro split. This leads me to my next point.

PREFERENCES

We all have different taste buds, and the amount of carbs we consume can also be boiled down to personal preference. Since everyone has a unique palate, some people love the carbs (like myself), and others prefer the wonderful sensations of eating a high-fat meal. Some prefer eggs and bacon for breakfast, while others love pancakes and Canadian maple syrup.

GENETICS AND YOUR CARB TOLERANCE

Another important consideration is how carbs make us *feel*. Each person's body responds differently to varying carb intakes. This principle is called *carbohydrate tolerance*, and on a basic level, it can be traced to our genetics and insulin sensitivity. Think of our carb tolerance as a spectrum.

On one side is the carb intolerant or insulin resistant folks who lack enzymes to properly digest, absorb, and metabolize carbs. If you're carb intolerant, you may experience the physical symptoms of bloat, energy crashes, indigestion, a foggy mind, or a less satiated feeling after consuming carbs. These people tend to feel better and can lose weight more easily if they stick to a diet with a lower carbohydrate intake.

On the other end of the spectrum are the carb tolerant. These folks thrive off carbs, feel a surge of energy after consumption, and can perform at peak levels cognitively and physically.

Likely, you're somewhere in the middle of the spectrum. Our carb tolerance isn't set in stone, however, and can change. As we get leaner and incorporate more exercise in our routines, for example, our insulin sensitivity can improve.[39]

There are a few different ways to gauge your carb tolerance. One way is to ask your doctor for a blood insulin test, but this still doesn't provide the whole story. The other is a more qualitative approach and involves running another self-experiment!

Determining Your Carb Tolerance Using John Fawkes's Experiment

If you're on the far side of the carb intolerant spectrum, you probably know it already. But if you're like most of us and sit somewhere in the middle, it's a good idea to test different macro splits and note the impact each one has on your energy levels, mood, and satiety. Knowing that we're all different, you can test out different macro splits in your meals to help you figure out what gives you the most energy, makes you feel full longest, and doesn't cause you any digestive or health issues.

Personal trainer John Fawkes has developed a great experiment (and graciously has given us permission to include it in this book) to calculate your carb intolerance that he recommends to all of his clients. He also believes that people should "do their own testing to find their personal optimal mix of nutrients."[40]

Fawkes's experiment is as follows: Under controlled conditions, you'll eat meals with varying carb/fat splits and then, after each meal, measure how you're feeling, your satiety level, and the impact on your mood by giving each meal a ranking between one and five. This is a controlled experiment, meaning that you'll want to keep variables like the time of day and the number of calories relatively consistent over the duration of the experiment.

I've included the experiment template in the bonus materials on my website (https://www.emilyrudow.com/findyourstride/resources), where you can log and analyze your results, but the following sections describe how the experiment works.

STEP 1: CHOOSE THE MEAL AND TIME OF DAY

Before starting the experiment, you're going to want to decide the time of day and the meal you're going to use in your test. If you eat three meals a day—breakfast, lunch, and dinner—then choose one. If you're doing the intermittent fasting protocol, perhaps it's the first meal after you break your fast. If you're only eating one meal a day (OMAD), well, you don't have much choice there. Fawkes recommends choosing breakfast for the experiment, as it "tends to take place under the same conditions every day." Regardless, just choose one meal and approximate the time of day to maintain some consistency with your results.

STEP 2: DETERMINE THE MACRO SPLITS
FOR EACH TEST MEAL AND PLAN YOUR MEALS

This takes a bit more legwork, but you're going to want to calculate different splits per meals. Don't get too hung up on the details here. To help you,

Fawkes and I have provided some example meals under each category. You'll want to split each of your test meals by low carb/high fat, low fat/high carb, and moderate carb/moderate fat, and then test each of the splits for *a minimum of three times.*

Instead of including grams, I've included percentages so you can calculate each split based on your own caloric needs and not your weight. During the experiment, try to choose foods that have nutrition labels, and use a food scale so you can properly measure out portions. MyFitnessPal and similar apps allow you to log the foods and portions in each meal, and then the app automatically calculates the macro split for you.

MODERATE FAT/MODERATE CARB

~15–20% calories from fat, ~45–55% of calories from carbs, and the rest from protein
Meal example: 4 oz. grilled chicken breast, 100 g baked sweet potato, 2 cups roasted Brussels sprouts (seasoned with 1 tbsp. olive oil and 2 tbsp. balsamic vinegar)
40 g carbohydrates, 17 g fat, 32 g protein
45% carbs, 20% fat, 35% protein

LOW FAT/HIGH CARB

~10–15% from fat, ~55–70% calories from carbs, and the rest from protein
Meal example: 1 whole bagel, 1 tbsp. peanut butter, with 1 scoop vegan protein mixed with 1 cup almond milk
57 g carbohydrates, 13 g fat, 35 g protein
54% carbs, 12% fat, 35% protein

LOW CARB/HIGH FAT

~40–45% calories from fat, 22–25% from carbs, and the rest from protein

Meal example: 2 scrambled eggs, 1/2 avocado, 2 slices turkey
bacon, and 1 rice cake
16 g carbohydrates, 28 g fat, 18 g protein
26% carbs, 45% fat, 29% protein

Note that the protein intake should remain consistent with each meal, since
we want to focus on just the fat and carb splits.

STEP 3: RUN THE EXPERIMENT

As Fawkes suggests, you should record each meal split three times, which comes
out to a nine-day experiment. If you want to go longer, that's even better! You'll
want to record the following variables: date and time, food, number of calories
per meal, and grams of carbs, fats, and protein. Then you'll want to record
some qualitative data and rank each of the following on a scale of 1 to 5, which
includes your energy levels, energy stability, satiety level, and mood.

Energy levels: How much energy do you have one to two hours after the
meal (a 1 being tired/sluggish and a 5 being ready to go do a workout)?

Energy stability: How stable is your energy for up to six hours following
the meal? If you feel a spike in energy followed by a sharp decline, you may
want to record a score lower on the spectrum of energy stability, like a 1 or
a 2. If you feel pretty much the same energy-wise up until your next meal,
you would then want to record a score higher up on the scale, like a 4 or a
5. If you record a 3, that would indicate that you do notice some changes in
energy, but not enough to make a difference.

Satiety level: Satiety is how full you feel after eating and how many hours
before you start feeling hungry. If you're hungry again within two hours, you
should record a 1. However, if hunger reappears after four hours, that would
be a 3, and after six hours or more you should record a 5. Just keep calories in
mind here, and Fawkes recommends a meal size of at least 500–700 calories.
If you're eating a light snack of 200 calories, that just ain't gonna cut it for
six hours.

Mood: Do you feel calm and happy or down and apathetic? Your mood
often correlates with your energy levels, so you should see some similarities

here. Fawkes classifies a 1 as feeling nonclinical depression. A 3 is feeling good but not great. A 5 means that you feel awesome and, in Fawkes's words, "bordering on hypomanic."

A sample chart is shown on the next page. For the sake of simplicity, an example of each split is shown for one day; your chart will show three days for each.

A quick note for women: Try to avoid doing this experiment a week before your menstrual cycle or during your cycle. A week or two after your last period ends is a good time to plan this experiment.

STEP 4: ANALYZE THE DATA

After the nine days are up, you'll want to find the meals that give you the 4s and 5s so you will have a general idea on whether you thrive on more or fewer carbs in your diet.[41] You will, as Fawkes puts it, probably realize you're pretty average and do best off the moderate-fat/moderate-carb ration, but you may find anomalies. I, for instance, thrive off a high-carb, high-protein, and lower-fat diet. However, some people are the opposite. Again, this experiment will help individualize the macro splits that are right for you. It will also help guide you to develop a nutrition plan to maximize your energy levels and, most importantly, make you feel good.

Takeaways

Carbs are not the enemy. However, carbs can be the enemy if you treat them as such. If you find yourself ingesting carbs in excess quantities or are incorporating too many refined or processed carbohydrates in your diet, you might end up cursing them after all. As you now know, carbohydrates is an umbrella term, and foods in this category can range from Oreo cookies to broccoli. Carbs will not make you "fat," but eating in a caloric surplus for prolonged periods of time will lead to weight gain, becoming a hindrance to your health and wellness goals. Your genetics do influence how your body tolerates carbs, which is why it's best to run your own experiment to determine the right carb split that maximizes how you feel and perform. If you do have higher insulin levels or elevated fasting blood sugar, a low-carb diet is usually the way to go.[42]

Date and time	Meal	Carbohy-drates	Fats	Protein	Calories	Energy level	Energy stability	Satiety	Mood
8/19/21 12:30 p.m.	2 scrambled eggs, 1/2 avocado, 2 slices turkey bacon, 1 rice cake	16 g	28 g	18 g	383	3	3	2	3
8/22/21 12:30 p.m.	1 whole bagel, 1 tbsp. peanut butter, with 1 scoop vegan protein mixed with 1 cup almond milk	57 g	13 g	35 g	495	4	3	4	4
8/25/21 12:30 p.m.	4 oz. chicken breast, 100 g sweet potato, 2 cups roasted Brussels sprouts	40 g	17 g	32 g	405	3	4	4	3

DIETARY FAT

Similar to carbs, dietary fat is another macronutrient that has caused much confusion among pretty much everyone. Historically, fat has been chastised, and then exalted, and then demonized, and then glorified once again. Ever since Atwater proposed that a unit of fat contains 9 kcal/g and carbs contain 4 kcal/g, it was concluded that fat could naturally cause overeating and the consumption of more calories, and therefore weight gain. Some scientists also assumed that dietary fat consumption directly caused the body to store fat, which turned out to be false.[43] In the 1980s, the low-fat craze became dogma and was promoted by the food industry, doctors, and even some governments. At this time there was a surge in popularity of "fat-free" foods.[44] A low-fat, low-calorie diet was claimed to be the solution for weight loss and a way to help prevent heart disease.

As discussed in the carbohydrates section, Dr. Atkins's low-carb, high-fat diet became popular in the 1990s. However, Atkins lost credibility because some of his research was flawed, and dietary fat once again experienced a precipitous fall. Only in the last few years has the pendulum swung back in the other direction—from low fat to high fat—with the popularization of low-carb, ketogenic, and fat-adapted diets.

Like the other macronutrients, fat plays many vital roles in the body. As outlined in the carb tolerance section, how much fat you want to include in your diet is really up to you. Research has shown that our bodies don't need as much dietary fat as carbs and protein to function properly. Unlike with carbs, there is a minimum recommended intake of fat you should consume in a day. But first, let's dive into the last macro and clear up any possible misconceptions about fat intake.

What Is Dietary Fat?

All types of fats have a similar chemical structure that forms a chain of carbon atoms bonded to hydrogen atoms. Scientifically speaking, types of fat differ based on the shape and length on the carbon chain. We also now know that fat is the most calorie-dense of the macros, ringing in at 9 kcal/g.

Dietary fat helps our bodies absorb vitamins and minerals, which provides us with energy. Dietary fat is also beneficial in the following ways: it helps with blood clotting, inflammation, muscle movement, skin and hair health, brain functions, and the building of cell membranes. Fats are also highly palatable—they add so much flavor to our food.

Types of Fat

SATURATED FATS

Saturated fats are defined as a type of fat consisting of single bonds between molecules. At room temperature, saturated fats take on a solid texture. They're found mostly in animal products (e.g., red meat, whole milk, and cheese) but can also be found in plant sources too (e.g., coconut oil).

Decades of research claimed that saturated fats were harmful for our health and that consuming too much saturated fat can lead to heart disease and other health issues. However, new research has emerged suggesting that saturated fats do not cause an increased risk of developing heart disease. One meta-analysis looked at 21 studies, during a 5- to 23-year time frame with close to 348,000 test subjects. The researchers studied the correlation between the subjects who developed coronary heart disease or stroke and their consumption of saturated fat. The studies concluded that there was no significant evidence to suggest that dietary saturated fat was associated with a higher risk of heart disease and that more research was required to make a conclusive statement.[45] On the other hand, several studies claim that saturated fats do lead to an increased risk of developing heart disease.[46] So this will remain a hotly debated topic.

Reducing saturated fats can indeed be good for our health if we replace them with the poly- or monounsaturated fat categories (which I get into in a minute), but not if you're replacing saturated fats with refined carbohydrates that are highly processed and full of sugar. Still, most health organizations recommend keeping saturated fat to less than 10% of your total daily caloric intake.

UNSATURATED FATS

Unsaturated fats have double or even triple bonds between molecules and take on liquid form at room temperature. Unsaturated fats can be broken down into two types: monounsaturated and polyunsaturated. Both types are essential fats for our body to function properly. Our bodies are unable to produce unsaturated fats on their own, so we must get them through our diet.

Monounsaturated fats have single carbon-to-carbon double bonds. Examples of this type of fat include olive oil, avocados, some nuts, pumpkin seeds, and sunflower oils. Some research has shown that monounsaturated fats can help reduce the risk of heart disease and can help decrease inflammation.

Polyunsaturated fats have two or more double bonds in a carbon chain and can be broken down even further into omega-3 fatty acids and omega-6 fatty acids.

Omega-3s can help improve parts of muscle recovery, reduce inflammation, and reduce the risk of heart disease.[47] Examples include walnuts, flax seeds, eggs, and fatty fish.

Omega-6s can help promote immune health and also help prevent blood clots. Examples include soybeans, nuts and seeds, and safflower and sunflower oils.

Poly fats are super healthy, and by including these in your diet while limiting saturated fats, you can reap the amazing health benefits. Plus, aesthetically, poly fats can give you fresh and glowing skin and hair. Now, who doesn't want that?

TRANS FATS

The last type of fat is the demon-that-will-possess-your-soul type of fat called *trans fats*. Study after study has shown the pernicious effect trans fat has on the body. Trans fats are a manufactured by-product of a process called hydrogenation. Manufacturers use this process to convert unsaturated fats to saturated fats. Now, why on earth would anyone want to do that? In short, trans fats help with food preservation, which provides a longer shelf life. However, the financial benefits for the companies using these types of fats come at a very high cost to our bodies.

Trans fats can increase the LDL cholesterol in the bloodstream and increase inflammation, which can increase our risk of cardiovascular disease, stroke, and diabetes. Trans fats are so bad for the body that they've been banned from several countries (Canada, the US, and parts of Europe, among others). Even teeny amounts of the substance can have destructive effects on our health. A paper from Harvard stated that for "every 2% of calories from trans fat consumed daily, the risk of heart disease rises by 23%."[48] The take-away here is to stay away from trans fats entirely.

The Role of Fats in Training

Fat is stored in our muscles and is primarily used by our bodies during low-to moderate-intensity exercise. In high-intensity exercise, our bodies' go-to resource is glycogen (from our *new* friend, the carb). But for low-intensity or steady-state exercise, our bodies primarily use fat as fuel. So, as discussed in the carbs section, it's fine to go higher on the fat and protein and lower on the carbs for lower intensity, but for high-intensity exercise (like sprinting or playing sports such as ice hockey and soccer), we'll benefit from a performance perspective by going higher on the carbohydrates.

The Crossover

There's a point of exercise intensity that we hit where our bodies make the switch from using fat as the primary source of fuel to carbohydrates and vice versa. This switch is called *the crossover*. If we start out with sprinting (anaerobic exercise), our bodies will draw from our glycogen stores, but if we're holding a slow jog (aerobic), the body will start to rely on fat as fuel. The main reasoning is that with aerobic exercise, oxygen is now more accessible to be used to "oxidize fat molecules."[49] When you're sprinting at full speed, breathing becomes hard, but when you're jogging or walking at a brisk pace, breathing is more controlled, and more oxygen is available.

The Effect on Body Fat of High-Intensity and Low-Intensity Exercise

There is debate on whether low-intensity or high-intensity exercise burns more body fat. Since our bodies dip into our fat stores during low-intensity exercise, doesn't that mean we'll burn more body fat with this type of work-out? It's the primary reason many of us do fasted workouts or exercise when our glycogen stores are low and close to being depleted. The short answer is no. One paper in the *Journal of Sports Science and Medicine* deduced that we must always keep in mind the "absolute kcal" that we expend during our exercise session.[50]

When it comes down to fat loss, once again, we circle back to the results of energy balance. We explore this topic in more depth in Chapter 10, but just keep this as a back pocket idea for now.

Fat Loading

Have you heard of carb loading? Many endurance athletes (including myself) follow this eating protocol in the days and hours leading up to an endurance event (like a marathon or ultramarathon). The hypothesis is that by consuming a large portion of your calories from carbohydrates, you'll maximize your glycogen stores, which in turn will give your body readily available energy that it is not extracting from your fat stores. If you are an endurance athlete or have run marathons in the past, you've likely come across this strategy. Before any marathons or ultramarathons, I always increase my intake of carbs 24–48 hours before my big race. I deploy the same strategy the night before a long training run: I try to consume a carb-heavy meal, usually of gnocchi, Oreos, chocolate, chocolate containing Oreos, and whatever other treats my tummy is craving that evening.

Have you heard of *fat loading*? I've been running for 14 years, but until I started conducting research for this book, I had never come across this idea before. The theory behind fat loading is that rather than consuming high amounts of calories in carbs, you load up on the fats instead. Apparently, consuming all these extra fats will "protect" your glycogen stores and increase intramuscular stores of fat, which in turn will improve fat oxida-tion. In other words, it could help improve your body's ability to burn fat, which will increase performance. There are two ways to do this. The first is called *acute* fat loading, in which you'll consume 60–90% of your calories from fat three to four hours before an event—typically in a single meal. The second is called *chronic* fat loading (a.k.a. the ketogenic diet, or low-carb diets), in which you'll consume most of your calories from fat five or more days before the event.[51]

So does the fat-loading strategy actually improve performance in endurance sports? Sadly, no. Studies have shown that fat loading has proven ineffective and can even hinder performance (if swapping out your carbs with fat). The most frequent finding showed that fat loading actually *increased* the rate of perceived exertion, meaning that endurance exercise and bouts of high intensity felt harder when fueled by high fat at the expense of carbs.

The Ketogenic Diet

I would certainly be remiss not to mention the ketogenic diet in a section on dietary fat. The ketogenic diet has been around for a long time—since the 1920s, when a high-fat, low-carb diet was used to treat epilepsy and control seizures. Recent research is now looking at some of the other benefits as well. The diet is high in fat, moderate in protein, and *very* low in carbs. People on the keto diet typically eat fewer than 50 g of carbohydrates a day (sometimes going even as low as 20 g per day), with a macro split that looks like this: 70–80% fat, 5–10% carbs, 10–20% protein.

PROS

People who make the switch from a moderate- to high-carb diet typically experience rapid weight loss for the first weeks, but this weight loss is mostly water. Research has shown that a low-carb diet can be beneficial for someone with obesity or type 2 diabetes. It can even help lower insulin resistance and improve and even reverse type 2 diabetes.[52] From a weight-loss perspective, many people on the keto diet also report feeling more satiated than those on a high-carb diet—which makes sense, given that the keto diet allows over double the kilocalories per gram than carbs and protein. However, this is also dependent on the *types* of carbs they were eating previously. We know that diets high in dietary fiber are also quite satiating, so take this statement with a grain of salt—or tablespoon of olive oil. By severely restricting your carbs, you're also forcing your body to use fat stores as the primary source of fuel, which again, can help expedite fat loss.[53]

From a performance perspective, some endurance athletes or trained individuals have moved to the keto diet. One study that put endurance athletes on a keto diet reported that initially they experienced lower energy in their workouts, but that energy later returned. The athletes also experienced improved recovery, reduced inflammation, and better skin. One big drawback of a keto diet is that the athletes did not have the energy reserves for high-intensity bouts. In other words, they could perform at a steady state fine, but high-intensity intervals were a struggle and a half for them.[54]

CONS

I would classify keto as a pretty extreme diet, especially for those who have stuck to a diet consisting of a moderate- to high-carb intake in the past. Moving 70–80% of your daily intake to fat can be quite the shock to the system. Many people who make the switch report the side effects of lethargy, brain fog, and sleepiness, which has been coined as the "keto flu." While these effects may fade over time as the individual becomes "fat-adapted," initially the symptoms are quite common.

Another big consideration when adopting a keto diet is making sure you're getting enough nutrients. People following keto can become nutrient deficient (in dietary fiber, vitamins, and minerals) because they do not eat enough fruits, vegetables, and whole grains. Constipation can also be a common side effect of keto because of the diet's lack of dietary fiber. Keto is also very restrictive and rigid, which makes it a difficult diet to adhere to over the long term.

The last big drawback of keto is the emergence of bad eating behaviors related to the diet. For example, some people on the keto diet increase their saturated fat intake to unhealthy amounts. Remember the Double Down sandwich from KFC that consisted of two pieces of fried chicken as buns and included bacon, cheese, and some other random creamy sauce in the middle? This bad boy clocked in at 37 g of fat (11 g saturated and 1 g trans), 18 g of carbs, and 52 g of protein. The sodium was off the charts at 1,880 mg (125% of your recommended daily intake). If you do try keto, I recommend steering clear of regular consumption of the Double Down (and the like) and limiting your saturated fat intake. In addition, ensure that you're hitting your protein targets of 1.8–2.7 g/kg of body weight.

If you're on the keto diet and it's working for you, then great, stick with it. If you are thinking of starting keto, I suggest conducting John Fawkes's experiment, so you can test the waters with a few high-fat meals.

Takeaways

We need a minimum amount of fats to help us function normally, unlike carbohydrates, which don't have a real minimum requirement. Dietary guidelines from the World Health Organization suggest consuming 20–35% of your daily calories from fat. However, as mentioned previously, this can vary from individual to individual. Since fat does play a vital role in the body, it's important to include *some fat* in your diet. Most evidence points to a minimum of 20% fat intake to ensure we consume essential fatty acids and fat-soluble vitamins.[55] If you want to increase your fat intake and find you operate better from consuming a higher fat diet, then of course you can up your fats!

KEY MACRONUTRIENT TAKEAWAYS

The main points to take away from our discussion of macronutrients are these:

- Focus on hitting your protein intake first and then splitting up your fats and carbs from there.
- Your fat and carb intake are highly individualized, so there's no one-size-fits-all solution.
- Use John Fawkes's experiment to see how different fat and carb combinations affect your energy levels, mood, performance, and satiety.

After running several self-experiments over the years, I've learned that I operate best on a diet that's high in protein, moderate to high in carbs, and lower in fat. While I typically only track my protein intake, when I do keep track of my macros (usually when running self-experiments), I generally see my split fall around 40% protein, 40% carbs, 20% fat.

Now that you have an experiment template, give it a go yourself. Take the information in this section and put it into action. Experiments can be fun, and you can learn a lot about yourself in the process.

MICRONUTRIENTS

When starting a new nutrition plan, most people focus on the macronutrients only, and micronutrients (vitamins and minerals) tend to go neglected. But our bodies need micronutrients too!

Remember that example I mentioned at the beginning of the macro section of the professor who lost weight from a diet of whey protein, Oreos, Doritos, Twinkies, and other highly processed snacks? So yes, the saying goes, "If it fits your macros . . ." I would also add, "If you hit your protein targets, follow a progressive training plan, and adhere to the principles of energy balance, then you can hit your body recomposition goals." But is this plan healthy? Should this even be a question? The answer is a hard no. These types of diets clearly lack essential vitamins and minerals. If we're deficient for long periods of time, this can lead to all sorts of health problems, including disease.

Have you ever heard of scurvy? Scurvy (a.k.a. the pirate disease) is caused by a deficiency of vitamin C (due to lack of fruits and vegetables), which can cause gum disease, bruising, hemorrhaging, and death (if untreated).[56] You can even lose your teeth. Yes, you heard that right, you will literally turn into a pirate (kidding) if you go for prolonged periods of time without consuming vitamin C. There's a legend that's been passed down over the years about a university student who consumed a diet rich in Kraft Macaroni and Cheese and beer who contracted scurvy. Can this be true? I couldn't find any legitimate sources to confirm, but I would say, yes, most likely since that diet would not contain any vitamin C.

While the information in this section should be ubiquitous at this point, for our general health and well-being we must include fresh fruits and vegetables in our diets. While micros don't play a substantial role in our body recomposition efforts, deficiencies can cause problems. If we're hitting all of the major food groups, we should be good. For vegans, however, supplementation (e.g., vitamin B12), can provide the necessary nutrients.

Keep in mind that micro means small amounts, so we don't need a lot of these nutrients in our diet, but we still need them. On a calorie-restricted diet, the most common vitamin and mineral deficiencies include iron, vitamin D, vitamin B12, calcium, vitamin A, magnesium, and iodine.

It is much better to get micronutrients from whole foods, but if you have food allergies or don't enjoy some of the foods containing the vital minerals and vitamins you need, then supplementation is a good idea.

Let's look at each nutrient's role and what foods contain it.

Iron: Iron transports oxygen to cells and makes up a big part of our red blood cells. Iron deficiencies are the most common in the world, affecting over 25% of the world's population.[57] Iron can be found in dark, leafy green vegetables, beans, red meat, and peas.

Vitamin D: Vitamin D keeps our bones, teeth, and muscles in tip-top shape and helps with calcium absorption in the body. Vitamin D is also referred to as the sunshine vitamin because when skin is exposed to sunlight, our skin makes vitamin D from cholesterol. It's a common deficiency, especially for us folks who live far from the equator. Many Canadians supplement with vitamin D during our brutally cold winters because of the lack of sunshine. Few foods offer this vitamin, but some do. The highest concentrations can be found in oily fish (cod liver oil), red meat, liver, and egg yolks.

Vitamin B12: Vitamin B12 keeps our blood cells and nervous system healthy and can help prevent anemia. This is the most common deficiency among vegetarians and vegans, as B12 is mostly found in animal products, including meat, eggs, and dairy. Some vegan and vegetarian sources, including nutritional yeast (my favorite), tempeh, fortified plant milk (e.g., soy milk), and other fermented foods contain B12 as well.

Calcium: Calcium is super important for strong bones and teeth and is especially vital in childhood. Hence the saying "Drink your milk so you grow up big and strong." Yes, calcium can be found in dairy, but it is also in a variety of other foods, including dark leafy greens (e.g., kale, spinach, bok choy), bread made with fortified flour, and some soy products.

Vitamin A: Vitamin A helps maintain strong bones, improves our immune systems, and helps with vision by producing eye pigments. There are two kinds of vitamin A: preformed and provitamin. Vitamin A deficiencies are more common in developing countries but less so in developed countries. In a paper titled "Prevalence of Vitamin A Deficiency in South Asia: Causes, Outcomes, and Possible Remedies," Saeed Akhtar and colleagues point out that the main reasonings behind vitamin A deficiencies include "economic constraints, sociocultural limitations, insufficient dietary intake, and [poor absorption]."[58] Preformed vitamin A can be found in fish, dairy, and other animal products. Provitamin A can be found in leafy greens, sweet potatoes, tomatoes, and carrots.

Magnesium: Magnesium is an important and often overlooked mineral. It plays many crucial roles in the body, including regulating muscle and nerve functions and providing structure for our bones and teeth. It may help lower blood pressure, improve the quality of our sleep, and support brain health. Magnesium deficiencies are quite common—especially in the Western world. While statistics vary, scientific evidence has shown that a large percentage of the US population is at risk of being deficient. One study indicated two-thirds of the population is magnesium deficient,[59] while another showed that approximately 50% of the US population is consuming less than the recommended amount.[60] Both statistics are very high and concerning. Magnesium deficiencies can cause some serious health problems and often go undedicated because of the lack of symptoms and clinical testing. Chronic deficiencies in magnesium can lead to high blood pressure, type 2 diabetes, and heart disease. Deficiencies can be divided into two types: frank deficiencies, with which we experience symptoms and can thus seek treatment, and subclinical deficiencies, which can go undetected by our physicians and regular testing. The reason for such high deficiencies in the Western world is—you guessed it—the Western diet. Magnesium is stripped away during food processing. Further, highly processed foods can actually deplete our magnesium levels. Common medications can also cause depletions in magnesium (including birth control, blood pressure pills, diuretics, etc.).[61] Depending on age and gender, the recommended daily dose for adults is approximately 310–420 mg. Some foods that pack a high magnesium punch include pumpkin seeds, chia seeds, almonds, spinach (and the leafy greens), cashews, and soy milk.

Iodine: Iodine affects our thyroid hormones and metabolic rate. It can be found in iodized salt, so because of the high concentration of salt in our foods here in North America, we don't typically have issues with getting an adequate amount. However, iodine deficiency is still common among the world's population, affecting over 30% of people in developing countries.[62] Iodine can be found in seafood, bananas, seaweed, and dairy products.

Paying attention to macros is most important for our training efforts, but deficiencies in our micronutrient categories can cause problems, thus hindering our performance. While there isn't a ton of research out there right now, one systematic review and meta-analysis showed how a micronutrient found in plants called *polyphenols* can help improve performance in our workouts.[63]

The main takeaway is this: I encourage you to eat a well-rounded diet containing all the major food groups to ensure you get adequate micros. When it comes to our training and making palpable changes in body composition, however, it's the *macronutrients* that we really need to pay attention to.

SUPPLEMENTS

I truly believe (and many fitness experts would agree) that you don't need any supplements to hit your body recomposition goals. However, there are some that can aid in your efforts. I personally don't use many supplements (and never have), but a few do make a regular appearance in my nutrition plan.

Protein Powder

Protein powder can come in many forms, but the most common types are whey, whey isolates, casein, and various vegetarian and vegan powders. When working through your protein targets you may find it difficult to hit your total protein intake in a given day. Protein powder is a quick and easy method to consume larger concentrations of protein with a lower calorie and carbohydrate price tag. However, protein powder isn't necessary if you're consuming enough quality protein from other sources in a given day. The best form of protein is from whole foods, as protein powders are heavily processed, but they can be a good aid if getting enough protein is a struggle.

ANIMAL PROTEINS

Whey: Whey is an animal-source protein that comes from cow's milk. This is the most common type of protein powder and usually the most cost-effective. Whey can also help promote satiety.

Whey isolates: Whey isolates go through an additional filtration process whereby the protein strips away most of the carbs and fats, providing an even more concentrated form of protein. Each serving contains about 90–95% protein and is a bit more expensive than regular whey.

Casein: Casein is another protein derivative of cow's milk. However, casein is absorbed and digested more slowly by the body. Casein is a bit controversial in its effects on muscle protein synthesis compared to other forms of protein. One acute (short) study showed the effects of muscle protein synthesis on whey protein versus casein versus soy. Three groups of men ingested 10 g of the three different protein sources following a resistance leg training session and at rest. Researchers concluded that the group that consumed whey protein saw a 122% greater increase in muscle protein synthesis than those who consumed casein (post-exercise) and a 31% increase over the soy eaters. The study concluded that both whey and soy helped induce muscle protein synthesis over casein both at rest and post-resistance training and at rest. This conclusion was perhaps due to the differences in leucine (an essential amino acid) content or how fast proteins were digested and absorbed.[64]

VEGETARIAN AND VEGAN PROTEINS

Pea protein: Pea protein is made from yellow split peas and contains all nine amino acids. It's one of the more popular choices among the vegan protein options, and studies show similar muscle-building effects compared to whey protein.[65]

Hemp protein: Hemp contains a high concentration of omega-3s but low levels of leucine and lysine (both key muscle-building amino acids).

Brown rice protein: Brown rice contains all the amino acids, but it's not considered a *complete* protein because of its low concentrations of lysine. There isn't too much research on brown rice protein, but because it doesn't contain a whole lot of lysine, it's probably not the best choice compared to the others.

Soy protein: Unlike brown rice and hemp, soy proteins contain all nine essential amino acids and are a great choice for vegans and vegetarians.

Vegan blended proteins: Some vegan proteins have a blend of pea, hemp, brown rice, and similar ingredients.

WHICH IS BEST?

If you consume animal products, whey isolates provide the highest concentrations of protein, but they are more expensive than whey. Whey protein is a close second choice, and casein is third. Whey can increase levels of satiety.

If you're vegan or vegetarian, you'll want to go for the powders that have all nine amino acids and are considered complete proteins. Soy or pea proteins are both good choices.

Creatine

Creatine has been around forever and is one of the most popular and widely researched supplements on the market. It's a substance that is produced naturally in our bodies and is commonly stored in our muscles and brain. Creatine supplementation has been proven time and time again in scientific literature to help aid in muscle growth, improve strength during resistance training, and increase energy. Creatine is also pretty affordable and is one of the safest supplements to ingest. When taking creatine, there's typically a loading phase that lasts around five to seven days, when you'll increase your creatine stores in the muscles quickly (typically 20 g per day). After the loading phase, you move into the maintenance phase, when you drop your intake to around 10 g a day. While there's some confusion on the optimal time to ingest creatine, immediately before or after exercise has been shown to offer the greatest benefits. One study showed that ingesting creatine post-workout was more beneficial to strength and body composition,[66] while other studies didn't see much of a difference. So it doesn't really matter too much when it's taken, but try to consume it close to your workouts if possible.

Caffeine

Caffeine is a widely used supplement that has a multitude of mental and physical benefits when it comes to our fat-loss efforts and performance in the gym. It can suppress our appetite; increase energy; improve mental clarity, alertness, and focus; and increase exercise output during high-intensity bouts. Caffeine has also been shown to increase thermogenesis in the body (allowing us to burn additional calories) and to stimulate lipolysis (the breakdown of fats).[67]

Caffeine can also help improve performance during endurance activities and during bouts of high-intensity exercise. However, one stipulation is that the effects of caffeine tend to favor trained versus untrained individuals. One study looked at the performance benefits of caffeine on trained and untrained swimmers. The study concluded that a particular level of training was needed to benefit from the "metabolic adaptations induced by [caffeine]."[68] However, if trained, using caffeine to improve performance in endurance sports is a no-brainer—it can be a highly effective ergogenic supplement to improve output. Some studies have shown, though, that to reap the most benefit out of caffeine, it's best to abstain for a week or longer (since our bodies can build up a tolerance—reducing the effects).[69] Caffeine can also decrease our rate of perceived exertion, which allows us to work harder without it feeling as hard.[70]

When it comes to the benefits of caffeine on strength and power training, studies seem to show conflicting and mixed results. Weirdly enough, it can positively affect resistance training on some muscle groups but have no effect on others. One meta-analysis looked at 27 studies on caffeine's effect on strength and muscular endurance. The study found that caffeine helped improve strength during knee extensor exercises (e.g., leg extension machine targeting the quads) but not on forearm or knee flexors (smaller muscle groups).[71] While several studies have shown more favorable results with the use of caffeine in strength training and power-based workouts, it once again comes down to the individual, so it is best to experiment yourself and observe your own performance with supplementation.

There's an abundance of products on the market today that contain caffeine, but most can be drilled down to caffeine that contains water (coffee, tea, energy drinks, soda, etc.) and a dehydrated form called caffeine anhydrous (pills, powders, and energy bars). Its dehydration process results in a much more concentrated and powerful form of caffeine. Some studies have shown that from a training perspective (especially with endurance and high-intensity training), caffeine anhydrous is the best way to supplement, as compared to coffee, for instance. However, when it comes to dosing, you need to be very cautious, as even just a tiny dose provides a huge serving of caffeine. In some powders, just a single teaspoon of caffeine anhydrous has the equivalence of 28 cups of coffee.[72] If you decide to use this type of caffeine, be very careful, since even just a small error in your dose can be highly toxic to the body and even result in death.[73]

The recommended dose (based on body weight) is 1.4–2.7 mg/lb. (3–6 mg/kg). Research has shown that, from a performance perspective, you won't derive any additional benefits if you exceed 9 mg/kg of body weight per day.[74] So for me, at 139 lbs., I should shoot for 195–375 mg per day, and rounding up, that would equate to about two to four 8-ounce cups of coffee. Since I've been drinking coffee for years, I've built up quite the tolerance and can go higher on the range but likely won't see any additional benefits in my workouts if I exceed six cups. If you're new to caffeine supplementation, it's wise to start at the lower end of the range and, as you build tolerance, work your way up.

Since our bodies build up a tolerance, it's best to cycle caffeine if you really want to derive the most ergogenic benefit from the supplement. Take one week off, and then incorporate caffeine back in pre-workout, for instance.

However, a recurring theme in this book (if you haven't noticed) is that everything is based on the individual. So it's best to play around with your own caffeine consumption and observe the effects it has on your physical and cognitive performance. In terms of timing, 60 minutes before a workout or endurance event is a great time to supplement with caffeine.

Even if you follow the recommended dosing, some people simply can't tolerate caffeine in even small or moderate doses (or at all). If I exceed five cups per day, I typically experience adverse side effects, such as increased anxiety and headaches. Other detrimental side effects of overconsumption include rapid (or erratic) heartbeat, insomnia, issues with digestion, and a big crash in energy, among others. While caffeine is a great supplement, it is a drug and stimulant, so it should be taken with caution.

The Truth about BCAAs

Branched-chain amino acids (BCAAs) are one of the most popular and also superfluous supplements on the market. What are they? BCAAs contain three essential amino acids that can't be produced by the body (valine, leucine, and isoleucine). Some of the supposed benefits are a reduction in soreness, muscle-building properties, and a decrease in exercise-induced fatigue. For years I took BCAAs because I believed they would prevent my body from burning muscle when I worked out in a fasted state. After educating myself, however, I realized that BCAAs are one of the most hyped supplements on the market and one of the least beneficial. The preventing-the-body-from-burning-muscle thing is a myth. BCAA supplementation can be in the form of pills and powders, but BCAAs are also prevalent in many whole foods (e.g., meat, whey and soy protein, lentils, brown rice), which makes it unnecessary to supplement. If you're consuming BCAAs for the presumed muscle-building properties, it's probably better to just consume a protein shake pre-workout. BCAAs ain't cheap, so if you're on a budget, you can easily omit this supplement. I still take BCAAs because I love the taste of the fruity flavors and for the caffeine content. I also like sipping on my pre-/intra-workout drink (made up of BCAAs and creatine), which, as mentioned previously, is part of my workout ritual.

Final Thoughts on Supplements

While this list of supplements is shorter than that in most fitness books, I truly believe that you don't need much supplementation to aid in the attainment of your fitness goals. It's also difficult to differentiate what's true and what isn't, because most writers on the topic either sell their own supplements or are affiliates of other brands. Protein powder, caffeine, and creatine are the only supplements I use in my training. I enjoy BCAAs because they help put me in the headspace to work out, and I enjoy sipping on them during my workout—perhaps for the placebo effect. How much you want to include supplementation in your nutrition plan is really up to you.

CHAPTER 8

Alcohol

Alcohol gets its own chapter because it has very different effects on our bodies than the macronutrients. Consuming alcohol has been the biggest culprit for hindering my fat-loss efforts over the course of my fitness journey. Alcohol has led to weight gain, stalled my progress, and thrown me off my workouts. Even a few pints at my ripe old age of 32 leaves me feeling drained the next day, with little to no energy.

As I get older, I've come to the realization that alcohol has never really added anything to my life. It has only substantially detracted from it. I don't know if it's because I'm getting older or because I've shifted to a more holistically healthier lifestyle, but every time I drink alcohol, I feel exponentially worse than I did in my 20s. I think this experience is something that many people can relate to; our tolerance isn't quite the same as it was during the "golden years" of partying. Even after drinking a beer or two, my brain starts to feel foggy, and nausea begins to set in. The next day, like clockwork, I feel overwhelming anxiety that lasts pretty much the entire day. If I drink too much, well, let's just say my hangovers usually last at least 48 hours. While I do enjoy the fast, euphoric buzz after the first drink, that feeling quickly fades, and I'm left feeling like garbage. While I'm not trying to be a fun sucker, I think it's important to uncover some truths when it comes to the consumption of alcohol, given its pervasiveness in society. One of the lies we've been led to believe about alcohol is that life just isn't as good without it.

Let's first look at the latest research on alcohol and how it may relate to your training and your body composition. If you do want to include alcohol in your diet, you can, and I go over some practices later to help minimize alcohol's damage on the body. However, it's important to note some of the pernicious effects alcohol has on our bodies and our minds.

ALCOHOL'S EFFECT ON THE BODY

From a physiological perspective, as soon as we drink alcohol, it gets immediately absorbed by the bloodstream and heads straight on over to the liver. Our bodies process alcohol the same way as they would if we were to ingest poison. That is, any other nutrients we consume are put on the back burner so our bodies can metabolize and eliminate the alcohol as quickly as possible. As soon as it enters the liver, alcohol is broken down into acetaldehyde and acetate. Acetate suppresses fat oxidation; in other words, it blunts our fat-burning process. One study showed that the consumption of just two beers inhibited lipolysis (the breakdown of fats).[1]

Alcohol is also a drug; it lowers our inhibitions and causes dehydration, and its addictive effects make us want to drink more. Because alcohol is a *drug* and not a nutrient, its main purpose is to make us want more and more. That's why it's so hard to stop at just one drink. Unlike proteins, carbs, and fats, alcohol doesn't suppress our appetites and leave us feeling satiated. In fact, it typically increases our appetites.[2] This can, of course, lead to post-drinking binge eating (which, I'm sure, some of us can relate to). After drinking alcohol, we lose touch with our hunger signals, and our stomach seems to be a bottomless pit.

While alcohol itself doesn't make you fat, the overconsumption of calories (from eating) while drinking can lead to a caloric surplus, which we know will lead to weight gain. Alcohol also has a high calorie content, at 7 kcal/g, making it easy to overconsume and put us in a surplus. One tall can of an IPA (my former favorite) clocks in close to 300 calories. You can see how even three beers puts you up to almost 1,000 calories. So you're consuming these empty calories that don't keep you full (and can even increase appetite), can make you lose your inhibitions, and lower your metabolism. We can clearly see the many strikes alcohol has against our fat-loss efforts.

Binge-drinking episodes are the worst for fat loss, but casual drinks (one to two) once a week probably won't have a huge effect on your progress. But remember that alcohol's full-time job is to make you want more, so let that be a warning.

ALCOHOL IN OUR TRAINING AND MUSCLE BUILDING

Another strike against alcohol is the effect it has on muscle protein synthesis. A 2017 study put physically active men through resistance training followed by cycling. The men consumed 25 g of whey protein post-workout while drinking large amounts of alcohol (eight to nine drinks). The researchers saw about a 24% decrease in muscle protein synthesis even after consuming adequate protein to stimulate muscle protein synthesis. The study concluded that alcohol "[impaired] recovery and adaptation to training."[3] So in layman's terms, if you drink large amounts of alcohol after a resistance training session, it can inhibit and slow muscle growth—all that hard work for nothing.

Alcohol consumed in large quantities can also lower testicular testosterone in men. One study that drew blood samples from men and women who arrived at a hospital's ER overtly drunk showed a 45% lower testosterone level in the men's samples. Weirdly enough, the women's samples showed an increase in their testosterone levels.[4] However, light alcohol consumption (two to three drinks) was shown to not have any significant effects on testosterone.

BEST PRACTICES FOR DRINKING ALCOHOL

If you are like the majority of the population and enjoy some drinks, there are a few ways you can include alcohol without sabotaging all the fitness progress you've made:

1. *Minimize your fat intake on the day you're drinking, and stick to eating just carbs and protein.* Since we know that alcohol inhibits the breakdown of fats, it's better to stick with the other two macros.

2. *Try to drink on rest days.* Drinking after training will inhibit muscle growth, so if you choose to drink, it's better to not train on those days. Again, wasted effort.

3. *Eat a meal with high protein and high amounts of dietary fiber before drinking.* This will keep you full and minimize the damage alcohol can inflict on the body. Food can help the liver break down the alcohol while also preventing you from getting too drunk.

4. *Avoid (or minimize) beer and sugary drinks.* Try to stick to dry wine and spirits with low calorie counts.

5. *Try to limit drinking to once per week or maybe twice if light consumption (one to two drinks).* Any more drinks than this, and your progress may be hindered.

6. *Track your intake (if possible).* I know this is a tough ask, especially when your inhibitions are lowered because the last thing you'll probably do is enter in the calories from each drink you consume. However, if you somehow have this self-control, then it will help you become more aware of the high calories you're pounding back.

OTHER WARNINGS

Throughout my 20s I would undergo "dry months"—abstaining from drinking for a month at a time, usually in January (December was always a heavy month of indulgence with the Rolodex of Christmas parties and festivities on tap). Each year the experience was kind of the same—the first few weeks were easy, and the later two more difficult. The last week was when I really needed to ramp up my willpower (which was conventionally running close to empty) and couldn't wait for the final day, when I could celebrate my accomplishment with—you guessed it—a beer (or several). However, since I turned 30, things have changed. Alcohol has kind of lost its appeal to me, and some of the applicable social situations involving alcohol (parties, bars, etc.) don't much interest me anymore. Perhaps I overdid it in my youth, or maybe I like feeling good and energized more often than not. As I'm sure many of us can relate, I've had some bad experiences with alcohol; I've done or said stupid things, acted like a fool, and felt the dreaded "hangxiety" and shame the next morning. From my own personal experience, drinking can be a dangerous game. Throughout my 20s I drank to excess, and when I became self-employed in 2016, I used drinking as a mechanism to numb me from all the challenges and struggles that were going on in my life. While it seemingly worked at the time, it made my challenges exponentially worst.

The main ingredient in alcohol is ethanol, which is a highly addictive toxic poison that, consumed in large quantities or on its own, can cause coma and death. Alcohol not only sabotaged my fat-loss and strength-building efforts but also hindered my performance, stole my confidence, made me lazy and stupid, and gave me so much anxiety—something I already struggle with sober.

It wasn't until my 30th year when I started cutting down on the drinking and abstaining from alcohol for longer bouts (two to three months at a time). When I took these prolonged breaks, I saw some big, positive changes in my life and my mental health. I was able to transform my body (building muscle and getting leaner), had way more energy in my workouts, approached my work with more positivity and enthusiasm, felt more creative, and had more motivation to pursue activities that brought me *real* joy and fulfillment.

At the end of 2020 and in the midst of a turbulent time in my life (and most likely everyone else's—we will not miss 2020!), I wanted a clear mind to set a positive tone for 2021. I set some pretty lofty goals for the new year (including writing this book) and knew that there was no way it was plausible if I upheld my drinking patterns even on special occasions. I couldn't afford to have a day go to waste; nor did I want to waste one. Since you probably know by now that I'm a big fan of timed challenges and experiments, I wanted to see if I could abstain from alcohol for a full six months, which is the longest I've ever gone without a drink (since turning 19, or maybe even before that).

MY SIX-MONTH ALCOHOL-FREE EXPERIMENT

In my 20s during Dry January, I would avoid any "tempting" situations, including meeting friends for meals/drinks, going out to parties, clubs, bars, concerts, and so on. Most of my month, in the dead of winter, would consist of a whole lot of indoor chilling and watching Netflix. In my 30s, I shifted this mindset and decided that I don't want to miss out on any of these experiences; alcohol didn't need to be the focal point of them. I wanted to live life like I normally would and run a social experiment to see if I genuinely enjoyed the activities I used to participate in or if it was the lens of alcohol that made those activities *seem* fun.

I think we sometimes underestimate the power of our minds and how they influence our experiences. If we don't think we're going to have a good time hanging out with friends or going to a party without alcohol, it becomes a self-fulfilling prophecy. We'll feel like we're missing out on a good time. Being the only sober one at a party can feel boring or make you self-conscious.

If, on the other hand, we go into the experience thinking we'll enjoy the company, the deep conversations, or the event itself (whether that be a concert, sports game, or other activity), we're more likely to have a good time. One shocking realization I came to during this experiment is that some of the activities I loved doing when drinking I couldn't stand sober. I had only enjoyed doing these things because alcohol was involved. Let's take attending a baseball game as an example. Sitting through a three-hour game sober is tortuous for me. I find it incredibly boring and realized that for me the whole experience used to revolve around pints. However, hitting up a patio with one of my best friends was a great experience. I got to enjoy some amazing appetizers and great conversation, and no alcohol was needed to enhance the experience.

When I first started this new sober lifestyle (pre-pandemic), I actually felt anxious showing up for "drinks" at a restaurant or pub and ordering a Diet Coke, or arriving at a party with a six-pack of sparkling water. I was worried that my friends thought I would be boring or that I would even possess a "holier than thou" attitude and judge them for choosing to drink.

The truth is that alcohol stripped away parts of my true self. When I was drinking, I wasn't as articulate as I am sober, I lost my ability to make good conversation, and on some of the foggier occasions, I could barely even remember the conversations I had the night before. I certainly wasn't a wordsmith when I had too much to drink.

When people find out I'm not drinking, they have mixed reactions, but predictable ones at this point. The first and most common reaction is curiosity. They wonder "why I was choosing to not drink when drinking is just so much more fun." The second, less common reaction is when someone starts trying to pressure me into it (or guilt me) or automatically goes on the defensive about their own drinking habits. This is the most irritable reaction to deal with. I don't understand why my decision to not drink is anyone's business but my own.

I'm not judging people for their choices, and choosing *not to drink* is a personal choice and not a reflection on what I think about other people's choices. I don't go around telling people that I don't want to drink as bragging rights on how "seemingly" great my self-discipline is. In fact, one of the main reasons I publicly announced that I was doing a six-month challenge was to mitigate any questions/negative responses from those around me when they realized I wasn't drinking. I could simply say that I'm doing a six-month challenge. After further reflection, I thought more about how weird this whole situation is, and that alcohol is the only *drug* where we judge those who *don't take it.*

What I have noticed, though, is that my true friends don't care if I drink or not. They enjoy my company because of me and not because I'm their drinking buddy. Connecting deeply with people I care about offers the natural high I crave without any of the negative side effects that come with drinking alcohol.

Alcohol consumption is so pervasive in our society, and by choosing to not drink, I'm aware that I'm going against the grain. While I used to care so much at first about what other people thought (I used to meticulously plan out my reasons and even devised a script that outlined reasons for not drinking when out in social situations), I've kind of stopped caring what people think altogether. When anyone starts to probe, I just shut them down. I've realized that if people are disappointed or don't want to hang out with me anymore because I choose not to drink, well then so be it. No love lost on my end.

I know for a fact that I'm much more enjoyable to be around when I'm sober rather than intoxicated, and I'm able to create more lasting memories and experiences. When most events or social situations involve alcohol, they can become a blur of sameness. For me, this couldn't be closer to the truth— my memories all kind of blend together when alcohol is involved. But the lasting, real memories that I hold close to me are always when the day/night doesn't rely on alcohol.

ALCOHOL'S EFFECT ON MOOD AND ENERGY

Since removing alcohol, my energy has become a lot more stable. I sleep better, I'm able to regulate my moodiness (with fewer outbursts), I'm more patient, and overall, a lot less anxious. I'm better at dealing with my negative emotions—truly feeling them and then subsequently letting them go. Alcohol simply numbed my emotions and dulled my senses. For example, after a breakup (one of the hardest experiences for me emotionally), I would go out to meet with friends for drinks to get my mind off my angst. While I felt better in the moment, the next day my anxiety would be off the charts and all of those negative emotions came flooding back, but this time even stronger.

Since I stopped drinking, I've become much more creative, been able to stick with the commitments I've set for myself, and even enjoy everyday activities so much more, like reading a good book, joking around with my family, or going for a midday walk in nature. This six-month experiment was a great experience. I realized that alcohol is not a magic potion that helps me relax, but rather, it's been a huge source of many of my problems. I no longer have to experience the extreme swings that come with the use of a drug and can deal with my emotions on my own terms. Feeling with my emotions fully (good and bad) and letting them pass through me has been a cathartic and liberating experience. While my goal was six months, I ended up extending the challenge and live this new alcohol-free lifestyle today. Over six months in, I rarely even think about drinking anymore.

FINAL THOUGHTS ON ALCOHOL

How much you want to include alcohol in your life is up to you, but as you now know, there is more to the story than just calories in versus calories out. If you've struggled with drinking in any way, I highly recommend reading *This Naked Mind: Control Alcohol, Find Freedom, Discover Happiness, and Change Your Life* by Annie Grace and *Easy Way to Control Alcohol* by Allen Carr. Further, if you haven't taken extended periods off drinking before, I highly recommend giving it a shot. While it does take a bit of time to acclimate to an alcohol-free lifestyle, the benefits are immense. The hardest part of my experiment by far was the social pressures, but remember that anyone who doesn't support your decision to not drink either isn't a true friend (drop them) or might struggle with their own relationship to alcohol. If you decide to drink, just be wary of the negative strikes that can easily stall or hinder your fitness goals.

CHAPTER 9

Bulking, Cutting, and Body Recomposition

S o far, we've learned how to calculate your maintenance calories, determine your protein targets, and figure out your individualized carb and fat splits. It's now time to put what we learned into action, which involves going through the phases of building muscle and losing body fat.

This is the time where you really need to think through what you want to achieve from a physique and aesthetic standpoint. Do you want to lose body fat? Gain muscle? Do both at the same time? Do you not care so much about building a muscular, lean body but want to trim down for health reasons and increase energy? One of the most common questions when it comes to building out a fitness plan is "Should I try to *build muscle* first, or *lose fat* first, or try to *do both* at the same time?" These "phases" are called bulking, cutting, and body recomposition. I'll quickly define each phase as it relates to building out a fitness plan.

Bulking is purposely eating in a caloric surplus with the primary goal of gaining muscle. If done correctly, the excess calories in bulking can give you more strength in the gym and also increase bone density. Bulking typically comes at the cost of gaining *some* accompanying body fat. If done wrong, which is often the case, you can end up with a lot of excess fat gain served with a side of sluggishness and lethargy.

Cutting is purposely eating in a caloric deficit with the goal of losing body fat. Shaving maintenance calories for prolonged periods typically comes at a cost of losing *some* muscle, but if done correctly, muscle loss can be minimized. Losing body fat can also give us more energy, help us sleep better, and improve insulin resistance. If done incorrectly or the deficit is too severe, you may end up losing a bunch of that newly formed muscle and experience low energy, mood swings, and crappy performance in the gym.

Body recomposition (or "body recomp" for short) is either eating at your maintenance calories or creating a *slight* deficit with the goal of building muscle and losing body fat at the *same time*. Presented with each of these, most people will opt for body recomp. Lose fat and build muscle at the same time? Sign me up! While it is indeed possible, the body recomp process can be painfully slow, especially in leaner individuals.

Bulking, cutting, and body recomp are each typically done in phases with the end goal of achieving long-lasting changes to your body with a steady gain of lean muscle over time while also minimizing the amount of accumulated body fat. I want to emphasize that changes in our bodies *take time*—a long time. Don't expect changes to occur in just weeks. I'm talking months and months, and even years. That's why it's so important, as discussed in Part I, to find deeper reasons for our training. And yes, I'm going to repeat my trite advice on the need to fall in love with the process. Seeing progress will indeed keep you motivated, but you also need to enjoy both your training and nutrition plan to be successful.

Now, let's look at how you can determine where your starting point should be.

BULK, CUT, OR BODY RECOMP FIRST?

Admittedly, the topic of which phase to start with as a new or seasoned trainee is a confusing and complicated one. A widely held belief in the fitness community (and one that I fell victim to as well) is that to build muscle as efficiently as possible, it's important to get lean and lower your body fat percentage first. This concept is called nutrition partitioning, or the *p-ratio*, which can be rudimentarily summarized as follows: When you gain weight from overfeeding/eating in a caloric surplus, your body is going to either use those calories to build lean mass (muscle) or store those calories as fat. So when you gain weight and most of the excess weight is in the form of lean mass, you have a high p-ratio, and on the inverse, if you gain weight and most is fat, you have a low p-ratio.

Gilbert Forbes first brought this issue to the forefront of the fitness community in a 1987 paper titled "Body Fat Content Influences the Body Composition Response to Nutrition and Exercise" (which was republished in 2000).[1] The research presented in his paper suggests that leaner individuals are more likely to gain lean tissue than fat mass from overfeeding. In other words, if you're already lean, the extra calories you consume are more likely to be used by your body to build lean mass rather than be stored as fat. However, Forbes's article has many flaws, one important one being that the participants who gained lean mass from overfeeding were anorexic patients who were untrained (did not incorporate resistance training). Further, Forbes's paper was intended not to be used in a bodybuilding context but simply to elucidate the concept of the p-ratio.

While debate on this topic is ongoing, a great 2021 article, written by researcher and pro bodybuilder Eric Trexler, titled "Should You Cut before You Bulk? How Body-Fat Levels Affect Your P-Ratio" helped shed light on the controversies surrounding which phase to start with. In his well-researched article, Trexler concludes, "There is insufficient evidence to suggest that losing fat will potentiate hypertrophy or improve one's p-ratio after a lower body-fat level is achieved."[2] So basically, if you think cutting your calories and getting lean first will help induce hypertrophy (build muscle) more efficiently than eating at maintenance or in a surplus, you'll likely be disappointed.

For practical purposes, the decision to cut or bulk first is an individual one based on preference, among other factors. An important consideration worth noting is that these three phases aren't just about eating. To see palpable changes in lean mass, you need to incorporate a progressive resistance training plan, which I discuss in Part III.

Bulking

The bulking phase is where many people assume they can just eat whatever they want in whatever quantities they want. "Bro science" will tell you that you just gotta eat more to get big. Ugh, stop. While you do get to eat more than you normally would while in this phase, in order to minimize fat gain, your surplus calories should be conservative. From firsthand experience, and most others would agree, it's demotivating to gain a bunch of body fat, so you'll really want to minimize your excess calorie consumption.

A bulking phase can last anywhere from four to eight months depending on your starting point, how much muscle you want to gain, and how comfortable you are with the accompanying body fat that is likely to come along for the ride. If you're looking at your transformation in a yearly time frame, the bulk phase will make up a majority of that time. You need to dedicate more time and effort to this phase because it takes a long time to build muscle and strength. Many people choose the fall and winter months for bulking, since we're not typically wearing a bathing suit in January—at least not here in Canada. However, you can start this phase whenever you'd like or create a work-back schedule based on when you want to achieve your longer-term goal.

Cutting

If you want to start by losing body fat first, then that's great. While there are many articles out there that provide an arbitrary body fat percentage to obtain before transitioning from a cut to a bulk, it's really about your own goals. If you're starting with the bulk first, you'll want to transition from eating in a caloric surplus to eating in a caloric deficit to shed some of that body fat and get a leaner physique.

The cutting phase typically lasts two to four months.[3] The goal is to cut until you've achieved your ideal aesthetic look (from a body fat perspective), and then you can either go through the bulking phase again or readjust your calories to maintenance to uphold the body you've built. However, unless you're a physique athlete or bodybuilder, getting to the single-digit body fat percentages for men or below 20% for women typically isn't sustainable.

Dropping our body fat percentage too low can have dire consequences on our mental health and can have additional repercussions, including big drops in energy levels, poor performance in training, and a potentially negative impact on our immune systems. For women, very low body fat can result in amenorrhea (loss of our period) and fertility issues. Personally, I never want to sacrifice how I *feel* for a "diet," and neither should you. Life is too short to feel like crap because of a calorie-restricted meal plan. Remember, the main goal of this book is to form sustainable habits and to help you build confidence by getting stronger and healthier, while also taking advantage of higher energy levels to devote to other important parts of your life. However, achieving and sustaining that elusive "shredded" look does come at a price. I've gotten my body fat down low but have obsessed over every single portion of food that entered my body. Food ran my life and stripped the joy out of everyday activities. Furthermore, some research has shown a correlation between bodybuilding and the development of eating disorders. One research paper concluded that about 53% of bodybuilders had body dissatisfaction, which correlated to eating disorders.[4] The point I'm trying to make is that it is essential that you keep checking in with yourself during this phase and practice self-care. While it's great to get a leaner and stronger physique, it could also increase your likelihood of developing obsessive eating behaviors. If food is running your life, it's time to reevaluate your goals. We'll touch on this more soon.

Body Recomposition

If you're a beginner weight lifter and considered "untrained," or grouped into the obese/overweight category, you can also choose a body recomposition strategy. Even if you're lean, you can go this route; however, it can be painfully slow and inefficient. Building muscle is already a slow process. So if you want to try to be as efficient as possible, gaining as much muscle while losing body fat to achieve your ideal body over the long term, it's better to go the traditional route(s). Body recomposition means eating at your maintenance calories—or in a slight deficit—while applying a progressive training program.

Bulking and Cutting: A Hybrid Approach

Switching between bulking and cutting is a balancing act; by eating in a caloric surplus every single day for months, your body fat percentage will increase and you'll likely begin to feel uncomfortable with the excess weight gain. On the other hand, eating in a deficit for prolonged periods can have metabolic and mental health consequences. So it's therefore important to vacillate between eating in a deficit and eating in a surplus while in each phase. If you're bulking, you may want to incorporate a short cutting phase, or a mini-cut, which involves eating in a caloric deficit for a few weeks to shed a bit of body fat. When you're cutting, you'll want to include refeed days and diet breaks (which we'll discuss shortly) where you'll bring calories back up to a maintenance level or eat in a slight surplus.

Let's highlight an example. Say you're starting with a bulking phase; you're following a progressive training and adjust your calories to put you in a surplus. You start to see muscle growth (great!), but you're starting to feel a bit uncomfortable with the excess fat that came along for the ride (ugh). You're still not entirely happy with your muscle growth and want to build more lean mass before moving to a cutting phase. So rather than go through a prolonged cutting phase, you may decide to do a mini-cut. You'll then jump right back in to your bulking phase and go through another round of eating in a caloric surplus.

Personal trainer Mike Thurston will do a month or two of bulking or eating in a slight surplus. However, when Thurston's body fat percentage creeps up, he'll do a mini-cut lasting two to four weeks to reduce body fat. Thurston will then go back to the next phase of bulking followed by another mini-cut. Once he's happy with his progression over a four- to six-month period, then he'll do a more serious, prolonged cutting phase (8 to 12 weeks long). The goal, Thurston says, is to "see a progression of lean body mass over time."[5]

There isn't one specific formula here since each phase is highly individualized, but this hybrid approach can be a good way to offset some of the negatives from each of the phases. Let's now go through the process of figuring out how to adjust your calories in each phase.

BULKING: ADJUSTING YOUR CALORIES FOR BUILDING MUSCLE

I think most people fit into the category of "I want to gain muscle, but I don't want to gain a bunch of body fat." With the exception of some power athletes who eat enough to feed a small village in a single day, most people can achieve minimal fat gain by adjusting their calories to a *slight surplus*. There's also been an association with purposely gaining weight as being "unhealthy" (which it can be). No one wants to gain a bunch of weight and feel like garbage. Some people eat enormous amounts of junk during their "bulking" phases and thus gain a ton of excess fat. Further, it will be difficult to make the switch over to eating in a caloric deficit once you're so acclimated to eating copious amounts of unhealthy (and oftentimes, delicious) food. That's why, during the bulking phase, you should focus more on nutrient-dense foods.

So bulking gets a bad rap for a reason, and people like me tend to stay away from this phase. Since I've never really gone through a prolonged bulking phase myself—and I'm not a physique athlete and don't aspire to be one—I can't provide insight from my personal experience. However, let's turn to the experts on this one.

There is a way to build muscle in a *healthy* way while minimizing the amount of fat gain. In a paper titled "Nutrition Recommendations for Bodybuilders in the Off-Season," Juma Iraki and colleagues suggest increasing calories about 10–20% from your maintenance calories, with a goal of gaining 0.25–5% of body weight per week.[6]

To figure this out, you'll need to do some more math (sorry)! To determine your weekly weight gain and caloric intake goals, you'll need your maintenance calories (which you calculated in Chapter 6) and your current weight.

Step 1: Set Your Target Weight Range

First, figure out your target weight range using the following formulas:

Your weight × 0.0025 = lower end of weekly weight gain

Your weight × 0.005 = higher end of weekly weight gain

EXAMPLE:

For my current weight of 139 lbs.:
139 lbs. × 0.0025 = ~0.4
139 lbs. × 0.005 = ~0.7
I'd aim to gain ~0.4–0.7 lbs. of body weight per week.

Step 2: Adjust Calories

Next, adjust your calories to put yourself in a positive energy balance:

Your maintenance calories × 10%

Your maintenance calories × 20%

EXAMPLE:

My maintenance calories of 2,234 (calculated earlier)
2,234 × 10% = 223
2,234 × 20% = 447
I'd want to eat in a caloric surplus of 223–447 calories per day.

Experts recommend that if you're newer to the strength training game and on the leaner side, you'll want to start at the higher end of this range, and if you're more advanced and already have a good amount of muscle mass, you'll want to aim for the lower range, which will help minimize body fat accumulation.[7]

Now looking at these calculations, I'd want to aim for the lower end. Suppose I eat an additional 500 calories per day. In that case, that would amount to 3,500 calories per week, equivalent to about one pound of weight gain per week. I know my body well and will accumulate quite a bit of fat in the process. If I aim for 250 calories per week, that amounts to 0.5 pounds of weight gain per week, in which I will still gain a small amount of fat, but it's manageable.

For the lean bulking phase, it's best once again to experiment with your caloric intake and adjust as needed. If you're eating in a surplus without weight training, you're going to be gaining a lot of fat. How long you want to continue this phase is up to you. When you're happy with your muscle mass and no longer want to accumulate excess fat or are starting to feel uncomfortable with your size, it's best to start moving on to the *cutting phase*.

ADJUSTING YOUR CALORIES FOR FAT LOSS

The goal of cutting, as we know, is to decrease our body fat percentage while holding on to as much of that newly gained muscle as possible. You also don't want to feel hungry or deprived all the time—the "diet mentality" is typically associated with eating in a caloric deficit or, as some put it, "starving myself to lose weight." Eating in a caloric deficit for prolonged periods of time can mess with your metabolism and can throw your hormones out of whack. As you move through this phase, there are some strategies you can apply so you don't feel like you're "dieting." These strategies can also offset the negative consequences of calorie restriction.

To maximize muscle retention while losing fat, you should aim for a caloric deficit of 0.5–1% and around 10–20% off of maintenance calories.[8] This largely depends on various factors (gender, metabolic rate, and a myriad of other factors such as current body fat percentage), but generally speaking, this is a good starting point for most. Setting a goal to lose 1.5–2 pounds per week is aggressive, where 0.5–1 pounds is safer and more manageable. It's not recommended to go over two pounds of weight loss per week, or you're putting yourself at risk of losing the muscle mass that you worked so hard at building. Plus, it's more likely that you'll throw in the towel if that deficit is too extreme. Your mood and energy levels will suffer dearly. Trust me, I've been there.

Let's once again get into the simple math.

Step 1: Set Your Target Weight Range

First, figure out your target weight range using the following formulas:

Your weight × 0.005 = lower end of weekly weight loss

Your weight × 0.01 = higher end of weekly weight loss

EXAMPLE:

For my current weight of 139lbs.:
139lbs. × 0.005 = ~0.7
139lbs. × 0.01 = ~1.4
I'd aim to lose ~0.7–1.4 lbs. of body weight per week.

Step 2: Adjust Calories

Next, adjust your calories to put yourself in a negative energy balance:

Your maintenance calories × 10%

Your maintenance calories × 20%

EXAMPLE:

My maintenance calories of ~2,234
2,234 × 10% = 223
2,234 × 20% = 447
I'd want to eat in a caloric deficit of 223–447 calories per day.

HOW TO HANDLE CALORIE RESTRICTION

As mentioned earlier, when you restrict calories (especially aggressively), you could experience hormone imbalances, lethargy, and low energy. Calorie restriction can even cause your weight-loss efforts to plateau. In addition, it can also predispose you to more fat gain once the deficit is lifted. In your training, chronic calorie restriction can affect your performance and make your workouts unenjoyable. In short, it's not a fun time. The following suggestions can help prevent the negative side effects of calorie restriction:

- Try to resist the urge to slack off in your resistance training. To preserve muscle mass while in a caloric deficit, you'll want to maintain your strength training regimen and still work hard at the gym.[9]

- When you're eating in a caloric deficit, it's even more vital to ensure you're getting your target protein intakes to preserve lean mass. Remember the range 1.8–2.7 g/kg states we discussed earlier in the book? If you're in a caloric deficit, it's better to aim for the higher range of this equation, and at a minimum try to aim for 2 g/kg or more.

If you want to get truly *shredded* at a competitive level, then you're going to have to push through physical barriers and deal with low energy. For everyone else (including myself), I don't think it's worth feeling like shit; nor is it sustainable to suffer for fat-loss purposes. Therefore, here are some tools you can use to help you in your cutting phase.

REFEED DAYS

Have you heard of the term *refeed days*? Restricting calories is a tough gig. It's even tougher to sustain over long periods. This is where the refeed days come in! The idea is to include some days during your cutting phase where you bring calories back up to maintenance or eat in a surplus to give your body a break from calorie restriction—making the whole ordeal much more enjoyable and sustainable.

A hormonal issue can arise when we restrict our calories. Leptin is produced by fat cells and is also referred to as the satiety or starvation hormone. Leptin's primary function is to regulate fat storage in our bodies. On a basic level, when we're eating enough, our leptin levels are higher and send a signal to the brain that we don't need to eat any more—giving the body the green light to burn the calories we consume. When we're restricting energy intake and when body fat levels are low, leptin levels are typically lower as well—telling our bodies to eat more and burn less energy.[10]

When leptin levels go down, our powerful metabolic forces may hold on to any of the last stores we have left, which can cause problems. Leptin tries to convince your brain to eat more by sending your brain hunger signals. While we can ignore these signals for a while, eventually, we're going to give in. The result? Regaining any of that body fat that was lost during the cut. This process of eating more food and burning fewer calories is called adaptive thermogenesis, which messes with your metabolism and tries to convince you to eat more.

So here's where the refeed days come in. By bringing calories back up to maintenance or in a slight surplus once every week or two during a cut, you might be able to bring leptin levels back up again, which would stimulate your metabolic rate. Your metabolism can then help you burn fat more efficiently. The additional calories you eat should be mainly from carbs, as they have the highest impact on leptin levels, as opposed to fat and protein. One study showed acute increases in leptin from refeeding (from carbohydrates) but only saw modest effects on metabolic rate.[11] More research is still needed, but a refeed day can be an excellent strategy to bring leptin levels up. In short, a refeed day can keep you sane during a cutting phase.

How Often Should You Include Refeed Days?

There are no set rules on refeed days, but most fitness experts recommend including at least one refeed day every couple of weeks. This is, however, dependent on your body fat percentage, gender, fitness goals, and so on. A good rule of thumb I found helpful was to break down the number of refeed days based on your gender and body fat percentage:

Body fat percentage	Days of refeeding
Men: 10% or more	Once every 2 weeks
Women: 20% or more	Once every 2 weeks
Men: 10% or less	1–2 times per week
Women: 15–20%*	1–2 times per week

*Most women should aim to have a body fat percentage above 15% to support reproductive and overall health.[12]

When I'm cutting calories, I typically bring my calories back up to maintenance once during the week and then eat in a surplus on the weekend. I don't go buck wild with my calories. I bring them up to a modest amount and enjoy some more carbs, which usually come in the form of pizza, or I just double up on my snack intake. Maybe even a bit of ice cream, or tripling my daily popcorn bowls, or both. The options are endless.

How Should You Adjust Your Calories on Refeed Days?

Once again, this is based on the individual, but you'll probably be safe if you aim to increase your calories by 20–25% or so (from maintenance). So my maintenance calories are approximately 2,234, and I would bring up my calories by somewhere in the range of 223–447 on my surplus days. Some people prefer to incorporate two surplus days, but I prefer one surplus and one maintenance. Again, it's really up to you. Ultimately, you want to be in an overall deficit at the end of the week. As I proved when calculating maintenance calories over time, the day-to-day fluctuations and decisions won't make or break you. Experimentation, my friends, is once again the best way to figure out what works for you.

A Note for Women

Women have another added layer of complexity when figuring out a nutrition plan, which is our good ole monthly friend, the period. The week leading up to my menstrual cycle, I have an insatiable appetite and eat in a surplus for consecutive days in a row. When I get my period, my appetite subsides, and I have no problems eating in a deficit. This is an essential consideration because it might throw you off balance, and it's the reason why it's so important to look at not just a day at a time but, rather, the whole week. You'll have more wiggle room to listen to your body if you follow a weekly plan, and it allows you to eat more on the days you're hungrier (from hormones, lousy sleep, or whatever). Then you can plan to bring calories back down on some days where your hunger has returned to a more normal level.

DIET BREAKS

Diet breaks are similar to refeed days but last for longer durations. The idea behind a diet break is to give our bodies a more extended vacation from prolonged calorie restriction. These typically last for a week or two instead of just once or twice a week for refeeds. Diet breaks can be planted right dab in the middle of our cutting phases.

Pro physique coach Paul Revelia recommends diet breaks to his clients by bringing calories back up to maintenance, bringing down the cardio, and focusing on recovery. He includes diet breaks as part of his "coaching toolbox" because "our bodies need a break."[13] While this strategy may seem counterintuitive, increasing our calorie intake can help with improving our metabolism and can even help us move past a stall or plateau in fat loss.

An interesting 2018 study on the effectiveness of diet breaks divided obese men into two groups. The first group was on a 16-week diet eating 67% of their maintenance calories. The second group was eating the same 67% of maintenance but included a two-week diet break where they brought calories back up to maintenance. The results were astounding—the second group lost 50% more fat with no loss in lean mass or a slowdown in metabolic rate. In a six-month follow-up after the study was completed, the second group saw 80–90% more fat loss than the first group.[14]

Diet breaks may be more beneficial for longer-term diet phases rather than shorter ones. For sustainability reasons and to help break through fat-loss plateaus, these can be implemented for psychological benefits but also to bring our metabolism back up.[15]

CHEAT DAYS

Cheat days and refeed days often get confused, but they are not the same. The main difference is that refeed days are controlled by setting how many calories you plan to overeat. Cheating, on the other hand, may take the form of uncontrolled or controlled and usually involves many servings of indulgent food. Cheating can also be associated with eating disorder behavior such as binge eating, so it's worth discussing this popular concept in a bit more detail.[16]

If you're going through a cutting phase and sticking to a meal plan that you enjoy, you might not even be compelled to "cheat" that much. There are a number of food swaps you can make to help trick your brain into thinking you're eating the real deal. Also, since we now know fat loss is achieved by energy balance, you can include some more indulgences in your everyday meal plans—which might help minimize the need to overeat on a cheat day or cheat meal. Just be cognizant of your daily protein targets and aim to be in a negative energy balance at the end of the week.

There are some outrageous cheat day videos on YouTube. If you haven't seen them, some fitness enthusiasts will eat 10,000–25,000 calories in a single day—it's obscene. While entertaining to watch, it's probably not a good idea to replicate such behavior. Cheat days can indeed sabotage our weight-loss efforts if we don't practice restraint, but if we instead have cheat meals and put some parameters on them, then we can include them intermittently throughout a fat-loss phase.

There are also a few downsides to cheat days besides just the impacts on fat loss. If left uncontrolled and driven by negative emotions, cheat days can turn into binge-eating episodes, causing us to feel guilt and shame from overeating, which can drive even more of the unwanted behavior. I've been here myself, and it's a dark place to be. Binge eating feels like you lose control and eat past satiety until you feel physically uncomfortable. I discuss binge eating in Chapter 11, but it's an important warning to consider here too.

So that being said, a cheat meal is probably a better idea than a cheat day. It can be used as a reward and can help rebut the feelings of guilt and shame from a psychological standpoint—helping you stick to your meal plan while giving you something to look forward to. Depending on your current fitness goals, you may want to include a cheat meal once per week (typically on weekends) or even biweekly.

If you do see a bit of weight gain the next day, remember that it's probably from water weight, especially if your cheat meals are carb heavy.[17] One single, bad meal is not going to ruin you. It's what you do after that cheat meal. If you mess up and eat something unhealthy, it's crucial to not chastise yourself. Just keep reminding yourself that you are in a long game. Mistakes are guaranteed to happen along the way. Just *enjoy* any slipups and move on!

RECALCULATING CALORIES
WHILE LOSING WEIGHT

When I first was trying to navigate the confusing world of calculating calories and macros, I had a big looming question, which was "When do I need to recalculate my maintenance calories as I start to lose weight?" Since maintenance calories are determined based on body weight, if I lose five pounds, wouldn't that mean that my maintenance calories change? The inverse is also true. If I'm trying to gain weight, how often should I recalculate as my weight increases? I was honestly so confused. Should I adjust it for every 1 pound, 5 pounds, or 10 pounds lost/gained? *Help!*

During my research, the answer to this question appeared to be overly complicated. However, I did discover a rule of thumb that was helpful. Basically, if you're starting to see plateaus in weight loss or weight gain while consistently training and eating your designated macro and calorie goals, it might be time to recalculate your calories. The fitness coach and owner of *A Workout Routine* known only as "Jay" suggests, "Don't recalculate or adjust any aspect of your diet until progress has consistently stopped altogether or maybe just slowed down to a significant (and unacceptable) degree. Basically, don't do anything until there's an actual need to do so."[18]

Jay recommends recalculating if you see a stall in your progress between two and four weeks. When you are moving along in your body recomposition journey, expect some stalls along the way. So it's essential to wait at least a couple of weeks before making any substantial changes to your calorie intake.

If you use MyFitnessPal to track your calories and macros and your weight-loss or weight-gain goals, the app will recalculate your calorie intake goal (based on what you input into the settings) for every 10 pounds you lose or gain from your starting weight. If you want to force a change in the app, you can adjust your original weight 10 pounds up from your current weight.

FAT-LOSS SUSTAINABILITY

Remember that cutting calories aggressively runs counter to sustainability. Instead of chastising yourself for losing less weight than intended or even stalling in a given week, just keep moving forward. We learned that as your body fat percentage goes down, the hormone leptin will try and stall your fat-loss progress. For prolonged periods of energy restriction, it can also lower your metabolic rate. That's why it's so important to do fat loss right—circumventing yo-yo dieting and the cyclicality of weight loss—losing weight, regaining, losing, regaining, rinse, repeat forever. Losing body fat is hard and it takes time. Practicing self-compassion as you go through this process is important. Just remember that if your plan is extreme (anything over two pounds per week) or you're feeling your energy levels take a turn for the worst, it's time to scale back—even if that means that you're not making progress as fast as you'd like. Let me repeat: sustainability is our goal here—shortcuts and extremes will likely leave us feeling miserable. Play the long game and foster some patience. It's worth it, I promise.

ADJUSTING CALORIES FOR BODY RECOMPOSITION

It is indeed possible to lose fat and gain muscle simultaneously, so going through a definitive bulking or cutting phase isn't necessary to achieve your fitness goals. The *rate* at which you achieve your goals depends on how lean you are, whether you're new to weight lifting (or coming back from a long training break), genetics, hormones, gender, even race, among a myriad of other variables.

Body recomposition is, therefore, the one phase that requires the most experimentation with several schools of thought. This phase contains all the shades of gray. I've had to play around with this strategy quite a bit, but what's worked for me is to eat at maintenance calories (as I calculated in Chapter 6) or eat in a slight deficit (I'd advise going lower on the range, about 10% off maintenance or even less). I alternate the two based on how hungry I am that day and how hard my training is. Since I'm a cis woman, my caloric needs also depend on my menstrual cycle. I get much hungrier in the week leading up to my period, so I need to at least eat at maintenance or in a slight surplus. Since there are so many conflicting opinions on body recomp, I asked personal trainer and founder of the popular YouTube channel Anabolic Aliens, Mike Rosa (who I deeply respect and admire), how he adjusts his clients' calories if they want to achieve body recomp. Here's what Rosa had to say:

> I would have [my clients] follow a caloric cycling method starting in a slight surplus to kick off their muscle building phase strong and energized, then end the plan in a slight deficit to aid the fat-loss goal throughout the same process. For example, if someone's maintenance caloric intake was 3,000 calories, then an approach I may take would be an initial 6-week caloric cycling strategy following a setup like this: Week 1: 3,400, Week 2: 3,200, Week 3: 3,000, Week 4: 2,800, Week 5: 2,600, Week 6: 2,400. This way they're steadily decreasing their caloric intake for fat loss as they follow a progressive training plan to gain muscle. Then I'd reevaluate for next steps after the first strategy is correctly and fully complete.[19]

This is a great strategy to pursue if you're new to training, as you'll likely see faster results with building muscle while losing body fat. However, if you are a veteran of training, note that it may take longer than going through a proper bulking phase.

CHAPTER 10

Nutrition Timing

N ow that you have a better idea of your nutrition and fitness goals—building muscle, losing fat, or both—let's consider a concept that can help you in those efforts: nutrition timing. It's about paying attention to the timing of when and what we eat, typically before and during workouts.

NUTRITION TIMING STRATEGIES

Improving performance in our workouts and optimizing energy levels are the main reasons why each of us should adopt a nutrition timing strategy. In Chapter 7, we looked at how each macronutrient plays a role in our training, but this section takes it a step further and outlines what to consume and when—before and during a workout—to help you run faster, lift more, and feel good. Once again, there is no one straight answer or one-size-fits-all approach when it comes to nutrition timing. You will need to experiment with different strategies that can help you determine which approach works best for you.

My nutrition timing strategy is in a constant state of flux. I'm always experimenting with new methods and tweaking as I go. I've devised some general guidelines for myself, but I've realized that as my body and workouts change, my strategies need to change too. I've found that one nutrition timing strategy might work great for one type of workout at a specific time of day (resistance training, for instance) but doesn't work for another (a long run). I encourage you to be agile in your approach as well.

Working out in a fed state or fasted state are the two most popular timing strategies. But which is better? Well, it depends. It depends on your individualized fitness goals, the type of workout you're doing and duration, your genetics, and any underlying health conditions you might have. Let's go through each in a bit more detail.

Fed Workouts

After you consume a meal, you can be in a "fed state" for up to four to six hours on average. During a fed workout, your body will allow you to work out longer and with more intensity than in a fasted state.

The fed state is what most athletes are used to, and experts have emphasized the importance of a proper pre-workout meal—but why? Well, in short, by consuming the right pre-workout nutrition, you can maximize your performance, while also repairing muscle damage post-workout.

A research paper in the *Journal of Clinical Endocrinology and Metabolism* demonstrates that eating in a fed state was more beneficial for longer exercise durations but not for shorter ones.[1] So, if you're planning on a long run or exerting a ton of energy in the gym (maybe combining strength training with cardio), a fed state might be the way to go.

However, it also depends on your own personal preference. Some people feel light-headed when they work out fasted, or feel that they don't have enough energy to push through challenging workouts. If you enjoy eating before your workout, then keep doing so, and experiment with different pre-workout macro splits.

Now let's discuss what to eat while working out in a fed state. Once again, it's dependent on several factors, including the type of exercise, the intensity, and the duration. For lower intensity workouts such as resistance training, fat and protein might be sufficient if that's what you prefer. For higher intensity workouts such as anaerobic exercise, your performance will likely benefit from more carbohydrates.

Eating carbs pre-workout can help increase your glycogen stores, and in turn provide you more sustained energy during your workouts. Carb-loading is a proven strategy that endurance athletes (including myself) use repeatedly to help top off their glycogen stores before a big race. This involves eating a carb-rich diet for one to seven days before race day. I've benefited immensely from the carb-load strategy during my organized races.

As discussed in Chapter 7, you might want to choose higher-fat foods for fuel if you're planning a lower-intensity workout. You can't really go wrong eating a pre-workout meal that includes a mix of carbs, protein, and fats, but it's always a good idea to go heavier on the carbs.

Up until 2019, I worked out in a fed state. I worked out in the mornings and believed the myth that if I didn't consume any food pre-workout, my body would burn muscle as an energy source while exercising on an empty stomach. So, based on this fear, and whether I was hungry or not, consuming breakfast pre-workout became a habit.

About an hour or so before my workout, I'd eat a carb-heavy breakfast of 400–500 calories (usually composed of oatmeal, yogurt, protein powder, and peanut butter), which would take me forever to digest. Sometimes I'd digest before my workouts, and other times (usually on the days where I'd force myself to eat) the meal would just hang out in my stomach. Once (and if) I finally digested, I found my workouts to be just okay—not great, not even good, but just okay. After years of eating this way (yes, it took me this long to come to this realization), I began experimenting a bit more with smaller meals pre-workout (for example, a protein bar, or a pear/apple with a tablespoon of peanut butter, or a protein shake and banana). The lighter meals made a *big* difference in my energy levels. It wasn't until March 2019, when I was driven by curiosity, that I really started exploring the world of fasting. I began experimenting with fasted workouts, and once my body acclimated (after a few weeks of slight hunger pangs), I began to realize the immense benefits that fasting had on my energy levels and performance in the gym. Let's go over the nitty-gritty of what a fasted state entails.

Fasted Workouts

A *fasted* state simply means that your body hasn't eaten for several hours (8–12 hours on average), but with some people, that time frame can be even more condensed. It really depends on how quickly your body can digest meals. The most common time to work out in a fasted state is first thing in the morning when your last meal was the night prior and you can sleep off the fed state. However, if you are a person who prefers working out in the afternoons or evenings, it is still possible to work out fasted by allowing your body a certain gap in time from your last meal.

Do Fasted Workouts Burn More Fat Than Fed Workouts?

Before we dive in to the real benefits, let's extrapolate a common myth: working out fasted could potentially burn more fat than working out in a fed state. Several studies reaffirm this finding and even conclude that you could burn up to *20% more fat* working out in a fasted rather than a fed state.[2] However, several of these studies focus on the immediate effects of the exercise session. While you may burn more fat during the actual workout, it doesn't necessarily mean you'll lose more fat at the end of the day.

A 2014 four-week study took twenty females and assigned them to two groups: a fasted training group and a fed group. They performed one hour of steady-state cardio three times per week while also following a meal plan that put them in a caloric deficit. At the end of the study, both groups showed significant weight loss (from being in a caloric deficit) with *no significant difference in fat loss or weight loss between groups.* Meaning that both fed and fasted training were *equally effective.*[3] So, while yes, it is established that fat oxidation increases after fasted aerobic exercise, over time, there doesn't seem to be much difference in body composition.

However, it's worth noting that there haven't been too many studies on the shorter-term effects of fasted training. But the main takeaway is that if you're only doing fasted cardio for the weight-loss/fat-loss benefits, it doesn't seem to matter whether you're fasted or fed, as long as, once again, you're in a caloric deficit at the end of the day.

Benefits of Fasted Workouts

Even though fasted workouts may not help us trim down the fat, there are many other benefits to consider when working out in a fasted state. The first issue involves digestion—it can be a lengthy process not only to digest your meals but also to use that food for fuel. After you eat, your body is drawing blood to help aid digestion rather than using that energy to fuel your workouts. When working out fasted, you can altogether avoid the issue of how much to eat and how soon before a workout.

From a performance perspective, working out fasted teaches your body to access different fuel sources. Instead of using glycogen, your body is tapping into your fat stores for energy. Working out fasted can improve fat oxidation in the longer term.[4] If your body can learn to better utilize fat, it could help improve performance in endurance events since we know that after the crossover, your body uses fat stores as its preferred source of fuel over carbohydrates. This may even give endurance athletes a bit of an advantage on race day. However, there isn't a whole lot of research to prove this; it's more hypothetical at this point.

If you're new to the fasting game, a quick word of advice: Like any adjustment to a new diet or training regimen, your body is going to need some time to adapt. You may have been eating before your workout for many years, so it's going to be a bit of a shock to the system. When I got back on the fasting train after a long break, it took around three days of fasted workouts to get my body to adjust fully. I found myself suffering from low energy one day, and then experiencing severe hunger pains the next day. Just be forewarned that it may take time to reap the benefits.

When You Shouldn't Work Out in a Fasted State

I would be remiss without mentioning a few warnings when it comes to fasted workouts. It's probably not wise to work out fasted for long durations, or during high-intensity workouts or endurance events. I've suffered too many times from what runners call *the dreaded bonk*—feeling light-headed and suffering through the remainder of the run because of insufficient nutrition.

INTRA-WORKOUT NUTRITION

Intra refers to *during* workouts. Depending on the duration of your exercise session, ingesting calories (mostly from a quick-absorbing carbohydrate source) can help reduce fatigue and extend your efforts. Aside from duration, whether you decide to fuel during your workout depends on the same variables: the type of activity, intensity, and how well you digest your calories. For activities where you're burning significant calories (for example, long runs), you should be ingesting some form of nutrition during your workout. For regular workouts, however, the decision to consume nutrition during your workout depends on each individual. With weight lifting, studies have shown that consuming carbohydrates alone or with a protein source during resistance training will increase glycogen stores and can also offset muscle damage.[5] Personally, I don't consume calories during my regular workout sessions; it's usually more of a hindrance than a help. However, if I'm doing a longer run (approximately 13+ miles, or 21+ kilometers), I'll incorporate some race nutrition in the form of gels or chews, or I'll stop at a grocery store en-route and grab a banana.

If you do decide to eat during your workout, a carb source that can be quickly digested is usually recommended (fruit, gummies, gels, etc.). Again, there's no tried-and-true formula. Take the information you learn and experiment. Observe your results, and revise if needed.

NUTRITION TIMING IN PRACTICE

I'm not attached to a single school of thought when it comes to using a fasted or fed strategy. I use a hybrid of both—each serves a purpose depending on the time of day I work out, the type of workout I'm doing, and how my body is feeling on that particular day. The following is an example of a checklist I go through when deciding if I should work out fasted or fed on a given day:

- If I eat a lot of carbs the night before (about 50–75 g), I'll typically work out fasted. I usually eat my last meal around 8:00–8:30 p.m.

- If my workout is within two hours of waking up, I'll likely work out fasted. If I work out later than two hours after I get up, I'll work out fed (otherwise, I'll be too hungry, and my workouts will suffer).

- If I'm planning a run for two hours or longer, I'll definitely need to consume both intra-workout calories and pre-workout nutrition to keep me fueled and feeling strong.

- I curb my appetite in the morning with coffee pre-workout and spirulina mixed with water. (Warning: spirulina tastes like a swamp.)

- Approximately a week before my menstrual cycle, I get very hungry. If I ignore my body's signals, I get moody and lethargic, so I tailor my fasted workouts around my hormone shifts.

In sum, a flexible nutrition plan is the best plan to have, and what works for some may not work for others. Experiment, observe your energy levels, and optimize, optimize, optimize.

INTERMITTENT FASTING

We're not going to go into a deep dive here, but it's worth mentioning intermittent fasting (IF) because of its popularity and the fact that it could be used as an effective tool to aid our fat-loss efforts. Intermittent fasting, in short, is giving your body a break from eating. The eating behavior of fasting then feasting has been around for centuries; this isn't a new concept.

You can fast for a certain number of hours in a given day or for full day(s) at a time. There's a ton of ways to do this, but a few of the most popular eating windows include the following:

- 16:8 (most common): fasting for 16 hours and eating in an eight-hour window. A popular eating window is between noon and 8:00 p.m.

- 5:2: eat as you normally would for five days out of the week, and fast for two days

- 24-hour fast: don't eat anything for 24 hours

- 36-hour fast: don't eat anything for 36 hours
- The "warrior" diet: fast for 20 hours, and then eat in a four-hour window

One of the biggest benefits of intermittent fasting is the relation to fat loss. Depending on which approach you choose, it may be harder to squeeze in enough calories if you can only eat during a small window of time. Many people lose fat through intermittent fasting because they eat fewer calories in a day, which is why it can be a great tool in our fat-loss toolbox.

Research backs up the idea that IF can help people lose fat. A 2020 systematic review looked at 27 trials and the effects IF had on weight loss. In all the trials, the participants lost between 0.8% and 13% off their baseline weight.[6] Recent research has also proved numerous other benefits with IF. It can help decrease insulin levels, improve insulin resistance, repair cells, and increase fat oxidation, among many other benefits.[7]

While fasting, I found more mental clarity, higher energy levels, and more focus at work. I tried a two-week 16:8 experiment (eating window between noon and 8:00 p.m.) in 2019, but since I do so much cardio and work out earlier in the morning, I found that the rigid eating window didn't work great. I struggled to adhere to the protocol for more than a few consecutive days. Granted, the two-week period probably wasn't enough time to allow my body to acclimate. I still incorporate 16:8 from time to time, but certainly not every day.

Fasting is not for everyone, however. Certain groups of individuals should not be fasting for extended periods of time, as it could be detrimental to their heath. Especially with cis women like me, IF may not be as effective as it is with men and can cause issues with our reproductive systems, including amenorrhea (loss of a period) and fertility issues.[8] Pregnant or nursing mothers, the elderly with chronic conditions, children, those struggling with eating disorders, or individuals with either type 1 or type 2 diabetes need to be closely monitored when adopting an IF regimen.[9]

Just make sure to not use my recommendations as a definitive guide. Instead, take the time to educate yourself outside this book if you fit into one of the aforementioned groups.

POST-WORKOUT NUTRITION

Now that we've discussed the pre- and intra-workout timing sections, let's dive into post-workout nutrition timing—another topic that causes much confusion within the fitness industry. I cover *what* to consume to replenish your resources, *when* you need to consume nutrition to capitalize on repairing muscles, and *how much* you need to consume to give your body the adequate nutrition required. Let's start by exploring the idea of the anabolic window.

The Anabolic Window

Anabolic is a biochemistry term and, as it relates to fitness, refers to the process our bodies go through to grow and build molecules. Resistance training causes tears in our muscles, followed by a metabolic process: muscle protein breakdown (MPB) and muscle protein synthesis (MPS). Following a strength training workout, muscle protein breakdown increases (a key component in muscle adaptation and increasing muscle mass). Your body uses protein to help repair the damage done in training. Combined, MPB and MPS can be a determining factor in muscle growth.[10]

The anabolic window theory proposes that you only have a specific amount of time, or window, post-workout to consume adequate protein to capitalize on maximum muscle growth from your training session.

There are two popular myths surrounding this theory. The first is that the window of opportunity is only 30–60 minutes post-exercise. The second is that in addition to protein, carbohydrates must also be consumed to replenish glycogen in the muscle, stimulating insulin and partitioning nutrients to the muscles. Basically, if you don't ingest protein within an hour post-workout, the whole workout is void. You were probably better off just sitting on the couch eating Fruit Loops in your underwear. Sounds silly, right? While there is indeed a window of time to capitalize on MPS and slow down MPB, that window is much, much larger than just one hour post-workout.

The scientific community's consensus, though, is that they don't really know what the real anabolic window is. One 2013 meta-analysis looked at 20 different studies on the effects of nutrition timing on muscle growth. The study refuted the claim that ingesting protein within an hour post-workout affects the optimization of muscle growth after resistance training. The researchers also concluded that "any positive effects noted in timing studies were found to be due to an increased protein intake rather than the temporal aspects of consumption." Basically, if you hit your protein intake for the day, you should be good. While this study does refute the one-hour window myth, they also mention that more research is needed to determine the actual window.[11]

Another study looked at the effects of ingesting protein before or after a workout on strength and body composition (body mass or body fat percentage). A 10-week study with 33 resistance-trained men concluded that there were no significant differences on body composition and no additional benefits of ingesting protein before or after a workout.[12]

While there isn't conclusive evidence, most studies suggest the window is several hours depending on when the pre-workout meal was consumed. A rough rule of thumb is a four- to five-hour window that also includes a pre-workout meal. So, if you eat your pre-workout meal about one hour before training and your workout lasts about an hour, then you'll want to eat your post-workout meal within four to five hours. The big exception here is if you train fasted. If you're working out in a fasted state, you'll want to consume your post-workout meal as soon as possible (preferably within an hour after your workout).

Should You Consume Carbs after a Workout?

Another popular belief (and I for sure fell prey to this) is that you must consume carbohydrates in conjunction with protein post-workout to maximize muscle growth. There was a time where I'd stuff a carton of chocolate milk in my gym bag and chug it back immediately after my workout. The truth is that the number of carbohydrates you consume after working out doesn't matter all that much—as long as you're ingesting *adequate protein.*

Research has shown that ingesting carbs and protein versus protein only post-workout have similar effects on muscle protein synthesis and muscle breakdown. A 2011 study broke nine men into two groups: one group consumed only 25 g of protein, and the other consumed 25 g of protein and 50 g of carbs. The group that consumed both protein and carbs post-workout did not stimulate protein synthesis or inhibit muscle protein breakdown any more than the protein-alone group.[13] Another 2005 study showed similar results, but added that carbs can be beneficial post-workout if you're not ingesting protein simultaneously. However, if you are consuming both, carbs don't appear to have much of an effect on reducing muscle protein breakdown.[14]

You, therefore, don't need to consume carbs post-workout to help with muscle protein synthesis if you're getting adequate protein. Still, if you're not consuming protein, then carbs can have a positive effect. However, consuming carbs and refilling those depleted glycogen stores can make you feel better from an energy standpoint. So after a big workout or an endurance event, I always opt for a post-workout meal that's heavy on the carbs.

How Much Protein Should You Consume Post-workout?

Is there an ideal amount of protein you should ingest to reap the benefits of your resistance training workout? In the same vein, how much of that protein can your body actually utilize in a single meal? Both are good questions that we'll approach from a muscle-building standpoint. For protein synthesis to occur, we'll need to supply the body with adequate protein post-workout to boost muscle protein synthesis while inhibiting muscle protein breakdown.

Research has shown the range of 20–30 g of protein to be ideal, but it's more important that you're getting your *daily* protein intake. A 2008 study by Daniel Moore and colleagues found that 20 g of protein post-resistance training was adequate to stimulate muscle protein synthesis. There wasn't enough data to suggest that ingesting 40 g of protein or more provided any additional benefit.[15]

Other studies concluded with similar findings where 20–30 g seemed to be the sweet spot. There appears to be a limit on the quantities of amino acids our muscles can use for protein synthesis. This protein "ceiling" is known as the "muscle full effect."[16]

A few factors that can influence your individual protein needs include lean body mass and age (as you get older, you need more protein) and the type of training you're doing.

When it comes to figuring out how much protein to include in each meal, it doesn't matter as much as whether you're hitting your protein targets for the day. There aren't any real long-term studies that I could find, but a weight calculation could be beneficial for a ballpark number. One study showed the range between 0.2 and 0.5 g/kg of body weight to be sufficient per meal.[17]

The most important takeaway is to try to ingest at least *20–30 g of protein within four to six hours* of training (this includes pre-workout meals). To optimize toward faster protein synthesis, it may be beneficial to space protein intake throughout multiple meals in a day. Still, if you're doing intermittent fasting, it's okay if you ingest protein in fewer meals. The key here, once again, is to focus on your daily intake.

CHAPTER 11

Eating Behaviors

I titled this chapter "Eating Behaviors" on purpose; I prefer to not use the word "dieting" because of its negative connotation. Dieting is associated with deprivation from a psychological standpoint, and that's not what I want you to take away from this book. While it is an intricate subject, for our purposes, we'll go through the two major types of eating behaviors that researchers study: rigid versus flexible eating patterns.

FLEXIBLE EATING

The term *flexible eating* is exactly how it sounds: freedom to choose foods and non-dichotomous labeling of certain foods as "good" or "bad," or in other words, giving all foods an equal playing field. The phrase "as long as it fits your macros" is derived from flexible eating. Flexible eating isn't a free-for-all: eat whatever you want, when you want, and in whatever quantities you want. There should be some rough guidelines in place and awareness of your food choices; just don't turn those guidelines into strict rules. "Flexible," as defined here, also means more freedom in scheduling meals and a more lenient timeline on your fat-loss efforts.

RIGID EATING

Rigid eating is also exactly how it sounds: strict timelines (losing fat as quickly as possible), dichotomizing foods by labeling them as "good" or "bad," and creating self-imposed rules to follow. I think rigid eating stems from fear—imposing such strict rules surrounding our diet is a way of protecting ourselves from weight gain and exerting some form of self-control. Rigid eating is binary—it's black and white and not a very nice way to live. Further, the dichotomizing of foods is rooted in racism. Fat-positive activist and powerlifter Kanoelani Patterson writes, "Diet culture is rooted in racism in multiple ways, from the ways people talk about fat bodies to the ways mainstream dietitians and wellness professionals deem certain foods 'bad' without considering the cultural implications."[1] I've followed rigid eating patterns for so many years now, and the consequences of non-adherence are immense. "Clean eating" can be grouped into this eating behavior along with other eating strategies with strict rules such as keto, Whole 30, paleo, and the list goes on.

FLEXIBLE VERSUS RIGID EATING BEHAVIOR

So, what does science say on this matter? Don't strict guidelines help us achieve our goals? Don't we need to be cognizant of every morsel of food that enters our body? The answer is no.

One study separated almost 55,000 participants into groups defined as flexible and rigid. The researchers concluded that the flexible control group was associated with better restraint, lower body mass index, less frequent (and severe) binge-eating episodes, lower calorie intake, and a higher probability of weight reduction over the long term—in this case, a one-year program.[2] Three years later, a follow-up on the participants to evaluate their weight-loss maintenance over the long term concluded:

> Subjects show a number of significant behavioral improvements, for example, choice of low-fat food, flexible control of eating behavior and coping with stress. Subjects who maintain these changes by the end of the first year have a higher probability of successful weight reduction after 3 [years].[3]

Another study examined over 100 women who deployed the same two eating patterns. This study concluded the same as the first: increased weight loss and maintenance with the flexible restraint versus the rigid restraint.[4]

The pros don't end there. Yet another study found that flexible eating results in lower levels of depression and anxiety.[5] Clearly, these strict rules run counter to our fat-loss efforts in the long term, which leads me to the popular topic of clean eating.

PROBLEMS WITH CLEAN EATING

What does clean eating actually entail? Does it mean zero processed foods and only whole foods? What counts as "clean" and what counts as "dirty"? The consensus is there is no consensus! What a plot twist, *amirite*?

No one can really agree on what clean eating means. Basically, a person will choose some arbitrary rules, once again, dichotomizing foods with labels. When I think clean eating, I think broccoli, chicken, and brown rice three times per day, which to me is so boring, bland, and nasty.

In Jeff Nippard's video "Why You Shouldn't Eat Clean," he illustrates the issues outlined above and makes a convincing argument that clean eating isn't the best strategy for fat loss (in the long term).[6] Nippard uses the example of how some people categorize sweet potatoes as "clean" but white potatoes as "dirty." This argument, however, makes no sense from a fat-loss perspective.

Basically, it comes down to this: the more foods you remove from your diet and label as off-limits, the harder it is to adhere to. Another downside is that if you limit or remove entire food groups, you can miss out on vital micronutrients, which can then lead to deficiencies. One study looked at the nutrient intakes of 41 elite bodybuilders and found that over 50% of the participants consumed less than the recommended daily allowances. Men were deficient in vitamin D, and women were deficient in calcium, zinc, copper, and chromium.[7]

Plus, you miss out on the wide variety of flavors that life has to offer: the special dinners with loved ones, enjoying appetizers on a night out with friends, and for me, just sitting with a box of Oreos and almond milk while watching RuPaul.

Rigid eating comes with the risk of entering into a dark hole. More serious problems are likely to emerge: eating disorders and highly dysfunctional relationships with food. One study once again looked at the rigid and flexible control groups in women and concluded that the women who deployed strict rules with their dieting reported "more symptoms of an eating disorder, mood disturbances, and excessive concern with body/size and shape."[8]

EATING DISORDERS

Obsessive restriction of foods and only consuming foods labeled as "healthy" is a phase I went through in college. I only allowed myself a "safe food" list and put restrictions on what I could eat and what was entirely off-limits. My safe food list included fat-free, sugar-free, low-sodium foods, and all the artificial sweeteners my little heart desired. Real healthy, right? I only allowed myself one serving of whole grains a day (bread, wraps) that had to be less than 150 calories. Oils, sugars, fatty meats, and alcohol were completely off-limits. While I did lose weight, the rigidity of my diet put me in a self-made prison. When my friends asked me to go out for dinner at a restaurant where the menu didn't adhere to my guidelines, I'd make an excuse that I couldn't go. This happened often. An exception was sushi because I'd get only sashimi and edamame, which I both labeled as "safe."

I was also working out like a fiend but not giving my body enough carbohydrates to fuel my workouts, let alone my day-to-day activities. I felt sluggish and moody most of the time, but I was "content" because I finally had the body I wanted. This was the sacrifice I thought I needed to make. Unfortunately, as I progressed through my weight-loss journey, my relationship with food got increasingly dysfunctional. I started replacing whole grains with inordinate quantities of carrots, and my skin even started turning orange from the excessive beta carotene intake. I was letting food run my life as I obsessed over every morsel that went into my body.

Recently, I discovered there was a name for this: *orthorexia nervosa*. Orthorexia is an eating disorder that's a paradox in and of itself: an *unhealthy* obsession with *eating healthy*. It entails a highly restrictive diet, "ritualized patterns of eating," and avoiding all foods believed to be unhealthy or "impure."[9]

Orthorexia is yet to be recognized as a formal eating disorder. Still, many clinicians have observed this behavior in patients and it's gaining more widespread awareness among the scientific community. While it's great to focus on eating healthily, there's a fine line; it can easily get out of control (which it did for me). Rigidity pigeonholes us into a box that's hard to escape from, and obsessing over food can easily take over our lives. Even over 10 years after I first suffered from the disorder, I still observe traces of it in myself. I still catch myself labeling foods as good or bad, and I still restrict myself from foods I really love. Even though I've loosened up a lot by educating myself, I'm far from perfect. Orthorexia creates a poor quality of life, and there's a likelihood you'll miss out on vital nutrients and life experiences (like exploring new places to eat when traveling). In addition, it's anxiety inducing, and slipping up even to the slightest degree can cause guilt, shame, and even depression.

You might be wondering why I recommend that you count calories and macros because aren't those rigid guidelines? Emily, you're contradicting yourself. And to that, I reply: Well, sort of. This leads me to my next point.

INTUITIVE EATING

In 2019, I published an article in *Medium* comparing intuitive eating with counting calories and macros. I assumed intuitive eating meant listening to your inner hunger signals. However, what I didn't realize at the time was that there was an entire book on the subject written by nutritionists Elyse Resch and Evelyn Tribole. One of my article's readers graciously recommended that I read Resch and Tribole's book, *Intuitive Eating*, to educate myself on the subject. In my article, I suggested that while intuitive eating or listening to your body works for some, it doesn't for many others. I failed to realize, however, that there were many more principles and context behind the lifestyle. So let's allow Resch and Tribole to define the term they coined, so there isn't any confusion: "Intuitive eating is an inside job—it's about listening to the messages of the body through interoceptive awareness. When you focus on weight, it interferes with the process of becoming an intuitive eater."[10]

Intuitive eating principles include the following:

- Rejecting the diet mentality (getting angry at diet culture)

- Honoring your hunger (keeping your body fed with adequate nutrition)

- Making peace with food (giving yourself permission to eat)

- Challenging the food police (non-dichotomizing foods as "good" or "bad")

- Discovering the satisfaction factor (learning to enjoy eating)

- Feeling your fullness (listening to internal "hunger signals" and stopping when you feel "comfortably full")

- Coping with your emotions with kindness

- Respecting your body (feeling better about who you are)

- Moving (shifting your focus to how moving makes you feel instead of on burning calories)

- Honoring your health (making food choices that honor your health and taste buds)[11]

Many of these principles align with my take on a healthy way to live. Where we disagree is their suggestion to avoid any sort of calorie and macro counting. However, I do see merit in wanting to lose body fat and gain muscle—to feel better, healthier, and more energized in our own skin.

As mentioned previously, before I tracked what went into my body, I would say 80% or more of my diet was composed of nutritionally dense foods. However, I failed to make any significant changes to my body composition. It felt discouraging—I thought I was doing everything right and didn't understand why I couldn't trim down on the fat and gain the lean muscle I desperately sought. However, when I finally started tracking my calories, I realized that I was eating in a surplus most days even though I was still eating "healthy" as arbitrarily defined by North American standards.

My sister is a master of portion control and listening to her inner signals. While she does eat healthily, she also indulges. The main difference between my sister and me is that she stops when she's full, but I don't. Psychologically

I need a big plate of food, or in other words, "high volume." Otherwise, I don't feel satisfied. My sister, on the other hand, can eat tiny little portions, and when she is acutely aware that she's full, she stops. I also eat out of boredom and anxiety and would say I'm an emotional eater. When I have to track what I put in my body, I'm more diligent with my portion sizes; I don't let things get out of hand.

I am a bit ambivalent because I do think in an ideal world, truly tuning in to our body's hunger signals would make a lot of sense. Eating what makes you feel good and energizes you can lead to better food choices. I feel like Resch and Tribole's *Intuitive Eating* doesn't dive deep enough into emotional and habitual eating. These types of patterns can be long established and are so difficult to break. We can also lose touch with our hunger signals—even when I'm mindfully enjoying my bowl of ice cream, I'm still going to want more—despite feeling full.

As you already know, if we want to make changes to our body and positive changes to our health, we need to have some sort of awareness of what we're consuming and the quantities. I do think it's important to incorporate some of the tools in the preceding chapters to keep you apprised of your food choices—at least for a bit.

TAKEAWAYS

A flexible eating strategy is the best one to adopt because it incorporates nutrient-dense foods that give you energy and make you feel good, but also allows you to include the goodies that you love. In the next chapter, I go through some food swap strategies to help limit feelings of deprivation and allow eating larger portions for a smaller calorie price tag. However, that doesn't mean that we can't enjoy our junk. Highly processed and junk foods become problematic if they govern a majority of what goes into your body and you neglect to include micronutrients. Remind yourself once again of this fact: Every fat-loss plan that's successful puts you in an energy deficit.

CHAPTER 12

Food Tracking and Meal Planning

P revious chapters cover specific nutrition strategies to align with three common fitness goals: bulking, cutting, and body recomposition. However, if we want to make changes to our bodies, we need to also understand the foods we eat and how much we eat. This is where tracking your calories (and protein) can come in handy.

Research has shown that self-monitoring can help us lose body fat; the act of tracking or food journaling alone can lead to weight loss.[1] Think about it: if you know you have to keep track of everything you put in your body for a specified amount of time, you're less likely to snack mindlessly.

While the thought of tracking every single food item that goes into your body sounds daunting, you don't need to do it forever (unless you enjoy it). A month or longer is ideal, but even a week or two can present a whole new level of awareness of your eating behaviors. Are you being too rigid or restrictive in your eating patterns? Are you consuming more calories than you really think?

When I was stuck in a long plateau (for years) in which I failed to make any significant changes to my body, I was so frustrated because I truly believed I was eating healthy. However, when I started to track my calories, I realized that I was overeating and not getting enough protein, which stunted my progress and sabotaged my fat-loss efforts. In fact, tracking my food intake alone was one of the biggest catalysts to help me transform my body.

Therefore, I highly recommend that you give food tracking a shot. It does require a bit of a time commitment and manual data entry, but there are ways to automate it (especially if you eat the same meals and foods every day with slight variations). Also, once you get the hang of it, it may no longer be necessary to track everything you eat.

So, with that being said, I've put together a list of a few of the top food-tracking apps, detailed in the following sections.

FOOD-TRACKING APPS

MyFitnessPal

MyFitnessPal has a huge database of food, and its features include a built-in barcode scanner that is intuitive and easy to use, shows calories and macro breakdowns, and allows you to create and save meals (super easy if you find you eat similar foods each day). The app also has some great photo journaling and progress training features. You can import recipes and check out the nutritional information at some of your favorite restaurants. Oh, and best of all, it's free! MyFitnessPal is by far my favorite app, and for an all-around tool, it certainly gets the job done. If you've tried MyFitnessPal and didn't really like it, there are a few more food-tracking options you can check out.

MyNetDiary

MyNetDiary tracks more vitamins and minerals (37 nutrients) than MyFitnessPal (20 nutrients), tracks your physical activity, and has a barcode scanner. You can select your type of diet, which includes calorie counting, low-carb, keto, vegan, or vegetarian. The app also keeps track of your weekly weight loss, target date, and source of calories (macros).

MyPlate Calorie Counter

Livestrong's MyPlate Calorie Counter allows you to set daily calorie goals and offers meal plans. It also comes with a big food database and barcode scanner.

Protein Tracker

All three apps listed previously will track your protein, but there's an app devoted explicitly to tracking protein only. The drawbacks are that it only tracks protein. But I like it because it's simple. So if you don't want to track your calories and everything else, Protein Tracker can make sure you're hitting your daily protein intake!

Spreadsheet or Food Journal

Some people prefer to track their calories and macros in a spreadsheet, even though, yes, it is tedious. I also like this method when I want to look holistically at my calories and macros over an entire week or month. I know YouTuber and fitness trainer Mike Thurston prefers this method as well as many others fitness professionals. Food journals, although analog, can be a good way to track as well. It's an extra step to transfer your calories and macros from your food-tracking app into your spreadsheet, but the payoff can be big. For example, if you sabotage one day (eating in a huge surplus), you can view the week as a whole and try to balance out your food intake on other days. It's much better to do this than to consider only a single day at a time.

INVEST IN A FOOD SCALE

A food scale is the type of scale that I can get on board with. If you haven't used a food scale to measure portions, an investment in this little tool is essential. I bought mine online for only $12. Not only will a food scale help you become more aware of your portion sizes, but it can also prevent you from overeating, which is particularly important at the beginning of your journey. While you can also use some rules of thumb (e.g., a serving of meat is equivalent to the size of a deck of cards), with more calorie-dense foods (such as nuts), a small overage can result in a huge excess of calories. This excess may cause you to overconsume, potentially putting you in a caloric surplus and sabotaging your fat-loss efforts.

That's all you need. A tracking app and a food scale.

MEAL PLANNING

Planning out your meals in advance can be a real help in ensuring you're hitting your calorie and macronutrient targets. Whether you want to plan your meals at the outset of the week or take it day by day, the choice is yours. Some people swear by prepping their meals in advance—bulk cooking meals, say on a Sunday, measuring portions, and sorting into storage containers. Others prefer to cook fresh. When I first started this practice, I would plan out my meals weekly but found that on several days, what I had planned I didn't necessarily feel like eating. So instead, I would swap out meals from other days and already know the calorie and macro portions. By doing this practice, I got a good idea of portions and calories in each of my meals, which made it easier down the line to eyeball portion sizes.

Meal planning has numerous benefits: it can save you time, help you make healthier choices, control your energy intake, ensure you're hitting your protein targets, and limit the number of choices you need to make in a day, since decision fatigue is real. In addition, knowing what you're going to be eating in advance can help you avoid grabbing the most convenient and, often, least healthy option that's driven by hunger and emotions.

I'm the type of gal who prefers cooking fresh meals, so I plan what I'm eating at the outset of each day (typically in the morning). Most of what I eat in a day is pretty similar (with slight variations), so I've pre-saved meals in MyFitnessPal, which takes a grand total of two minutes to log. If you're one of those time-scarce people, there's also an abundance of meal-planning services that include the macros and calorie counts in each of their dishes.

You, of course, don't need to go the meal-planning route, but when you're first starting on a new nutrition plan, this practice can exponentially increase your chances of success. Research has shown that planning meals ahead of time can help you eat healthier, lose fat, and can be especially helpful in losing weight for the obese population.[2]

The following are my tips to start meal planning successfully:

- If you're new to meal planning, start small and plan out a few meals per day to get into the habit. Going big right away and planning everything might feel too overwhelming.

- Include a variety of nutrient-dense foods, but also make sure to include foods you love!

- Bulk buy your staples—for me, that's egg whites, Greek yogurt, almond milk, and protein powder.

- Track your meals in an app to get an idea of calories and macros.

- Go to the grocery store on a full stomach and with a list.

- Use a food scale to weigh portions.

- Variety is the spice of life (try different seasonings, spices, and so on).

- You can also use the nontracking approach, but that requires more consistency with meals.

Whatever method you choose, by planning out your meals in advance, you're exponentially increasing your chance of success. I'm going to be real with you: it is a bit of work, but it is well worth the time investment.

EATING FOR FAT LOSS (DEFICIT)

When you're trying to lose fat and eating in a deficit, hunger can and probably will occur. That's why it's so important to eat foods that are more satiating to keep you fuller for longer. Focus on your protein intake first, and now that you understand the math (I hope), you want to follow your daily calorie targets (shaving no more than 20% off your maintenance calories). With every meal you plan, try to incorporate at least one source of protein (remember the thermic effect) as well as foods with high dietary fiber. The strategy that's worked best for me is making food swaps. That is, choosing my favorite calorie-dense foods and making healthier replacements.

An important caveat is this: as I mentioned from the outset of the book, I'm a cisgender white woman and eat a predominantly North American–based diet with many foods predominant in the European diet. However, it's worth noting that some of these foods don't "burn as efficiently" in the descendants of people from Asia, Africa, and other parts of the world, as one study pointed out.[3] There are real genetic and racial differences when it comes to fat loss, so again, it's important to experiment for yourself.

In a similar vein, there is a lack of controlled studies with ethnic/minority subgroup participants in behavioral weight-loss interventions. One paper looked at 94 studies across PubMed, PsycInfo, Medline, and CINAHL, and concluded that approximately 60% of the participants were white, "18.2% were African American, 8.7% were Hispanic/Latino, 5.0% were Asian and 1.0% were Native Americans. An additional 8.2% were categorized as 'Other.' Nine out of the 94 exclusively included minority samples."[4] I think we'd be remiss if we didn't ask researchers why they weren't actively seeking out more diversity when recruiting participants in their studies. It's important to note that these studies aren't reflective of the diversity of the population, and therefore can't be used as a measure of truth among all individuals.

Let's highlight a couple of my favorite food swaps:

Regular blueberry pancakes (1 serving)	Protein blueberry pancakes (2 servings)
1/3 cup pancake mix (~47 g) 1 egg 1 tbsp. vegetable oil 3/4 cup 2% milk 1/2 cup blueberries 1 tbsp. butter 3 tbsp. regular maple syrup	2 scoops vegan protein powder (Beyond Yourself vanilla cupcake batter flavor) 1 cup egg whites 1 tsp. olive oil 1/2 cup blueberries 3 tbsp. no-sugar-added maple syrup

Calories: 548 Protein: 8.2 g Fat: 20 g Carbohydrates: 82 g Sugar: 51 g	Calories: 427 Protein: 66 g Fat: 8 g Carbohydrates: 21 g Sugar: 15 g

Poached eggs and avocado on toast	Poached eggs and avocado on rice cakes
2 poached eggs 1 medium avocado 2 slices whole wheat bread	2 poached eggs 1/2 avocado 2 rice cakes, tomato and basil flavor
Calories: 563 Protein: 23 g Fat: 34 g Carbohydrates: 46 g Sugar: 4 g	Calories: 363 Protein: 14 g Fat: 25 g Carbohydrates: 23 g Sugar: 2 g

Making a swap from regular pancakes to protein pancakes saves you 121 calories while increasing your protein by 58 g. In the second example, by swapping whole-wheat bread for rice cakes and having half an avocado instead of a whole one, you're saving 200 calories. While these differences don't seem like a lot, 100–200 calories saved from a single meal can be a big driver in putting you in a caloric deficit. If you make a bunch of swaps like this throughout the day, you're much more likely to hit your calorie goals while remaining satiated.

EATING FOR BUILDING MUSCLE (SURPLUS)

When you're trying to eat in a surplus to gain muscle, it may be tricky to eat so much food (especially if you're not used to it). That's why you'll want to focus on more calorie-dense foods rather than foods higher on the satiety index. Don't be mistaken—I'm not saying to *not eat your veggies*. I'm simply saying that you should try and incorporate more foods like oils and nuts to help bump up your calorie intake. Rice is typically less satiating than baked potatoes, and adding a few tablespoons of peanut butter to your oatmeal can bump up your meal by 200 calories. Historically, the bulking phase meant that you could eat as much garbage as you wanted and basically get fat. Don't do this. Of course, you can include some processed foods in your diet, but focus on the foods chock full of nutrients to make you feel your best. I like the good ole 80/20 rule, which is 80% of the foods I eat have nutrients, and the other 20% can be whatever I want. Popcorn and snack bowls with a wide array of processed chips are my usual go-tos.

A FULL DAY OF EATING

Let me just start by saying, I love binge watching "What I Eat in a Day" videos on YouTube from fitness peeps; whether that's bodybuilders, powerlifters, runners, or vegan athletes, I love all of it. I thought it would be fun, therefore, to include a few "what I eat in a day" examples in the following pages to give you a depiction of what I typically eat when aiming for a caloric deficit and a surplus along with the macro/calorie breakdowns.

In addition, in the Resources section, you will find sample meal plans at different calorie goals (1,800 calories, 2,500 calories, 3,000 calories), as well as vegetarian and vegan options.

A day of eating in a caloric deficit

2,183 calories, 154 g protein, 252 g carbs, 91 g fat	
421 calories 45 g protein 63 g carbs 11 g fat	*Meal 1: Breakfast (protein pancakes)* • 1/2 cup mashed banana • 1 scoop Vega chocolate protein powder • 1/4 cup liquid egg whites (bought in cartons) • 2 tbsp. unsweetened almond milk • Topped with 3/4 cup plain Greek yogurt, warmed blueberries, and 1 packet stevia • 2 cups raw broccoli
376 calories 25 g protein 27 g carbs 20 g fat	*Meal 2: Lunch (open-faced sandwich with low carbs)* • 2 mini rice cakes (tomato basil flavor) • 1/2 avocado • 2 oz. deli turkey • Protein shake: 1 cup unsweetened almond milk, 1/2 cup whey isolate protein powder, and 1 cup frozen spinach • 2 cups raw broccoli
570 calories 9 g protein 71 g carbs 30 g fat	*Meal 3: Snack* • 3 servings Skinny Pop popcorn (150 cals/serving) • 1 cup baby carrots • 1 cup cucumbers
457 calories 39 g protein 41 g carbs 21 g fat	*Meal 4: Dinner* • Zucchini noodles with Trader Joe's Chili Lime seasoning • 5 oz. chicken breast with chili garlic sauce • Roasted lemon potatoes with 1 tbsp. olive oil • Protein shake: 1 cup unsweetened almond milk, 1/2 cup whey isolate protein powder, and 1 cup frozen spinach
359 calories 36 g protein 50 g carbs 9 g fat	*Meal 5: Dessert bowl* • 1/2 cup heated strawberries • 1/3 cup Greek yogurt • 1/2 scoop whey isolate (Beyond Yourself cookie dough ice cream flavor) • 1 tbsp. peanut butter • 1/2 pear

A day of eating in a caloric deficit (vegetarian)

1,958 calories, 158 g protein, 197 g carbs, 71 g fat	
536 calories 60 g protein 38 g carbs 18 g fat	*Meal 1: Breakfast (blueberry protein pancakes)* • 1 scoop Vega Sport protein powder • 3/4 cup liquid egg whites • 1/4 cup unsweetened almond milk • 1/2 cup blueberries • Topped with 1 tbsp. peanut butter, 1 cup no-sugar-added chocolate pudding, 1 tbsp. pumpkin seeds, and 3 tbsp. no-sugar-added maple syrup
634 calories 39 g protein 73 g carbs 28 g fat	*Meal 2: Lunch* • 2 poached eggs • 1 cup vegetarian quinoa chili • 1 cup raw broccoli • 1/2 avocado (mashed) • 100 g tempeh (smoky bacon flavor)
366 calories 38 g protein 21 g carbs 14 g fat	*Meal 3: Snack* • 1 serving (~4 cups) coconut oil popcorn topped with 1 tbsp. nutritional yeast • Spirulina protein smoothie: 1 tbsp. powdered spirulina, 1 cup unsweetened almond milk, 1 scoop Beyond Yourself whey isolate protein powder (chocolate peanut butter flavor)
422 calories 21 g protein 65 g carbs 11 g fat	*Meal 4: Dinner* • 100 g tofu (seasoned with roasted garlic and peppers seasoning) • 2 cups broccoli • 1/2 cup coconut basmati rice • 1 cup mango

A day of eating in a caloric surplus (vegetarian)

2,446 calories, 185 g protein, 201 g carbs, 109 g fat	
567 calories 70 g protein 25 g carbs 21 g fat	*Meal 1: Breakfast (blueberry protein pancakes)* • 2 scoops Beyond Yourself vegan protein powder (vanilla cupcake batter flavor) • 1 cup liquid egg whites • 1/2 cup blueberries • 1 oz. walnuts and 3 tbsp. no-sugar-added maple syrup
255 calories 21 g protein 18 g carbs 12 g fat	*Meal 2: Snack* • Carb Killa cookie dough protein bar • Coffee with almond milk
434 calories 17 g protein 24 g carbs 38 g fat	*Meal 3: Lunch* • 2 poached eggs • 1 whole small avocado • 2 mini rice cakes (tomato and basil flavor) • Raw broccoli and cucumber • Sauteed mushrooms and red pepper
330 calories 13 g protein 33 g carbs 18 g fat	*Meal 4: Snack* • 6 cups coconut oil popcorn • 2 tbsp. spirulina with water and bit of stevia (*warning: this tastes like sewage*)
451 calories 30 g protein 62 g carbs 8 g fat	*Meal 5: Dinner* • 1 Yves Veggie Breaded Chick'n Burger • 1 baked sweet potato • 2 cups broccoli and 2 cups mushrooms • 2 tbsp tzatziki
409 calories 34 g protein 39 g carbs 12 g fat	*Meal 6: Dessert bowl* • 1 cup cottage cheese • 1 cup mango • 2 tbsp. walnuts • 1 tbsp. chia seeds

PART III

TRAINING

CHAPTER 13

Training Fundamentals

Back in 2008, when I first started lifting weights, I learned a handful of exercises for each body part from who knows where. I did a quick Google search on the ideal rep and set range and then got to work. Over the following weeks, I started to see some real palpable changes in my body composition, but those changes kind of tapered off over subsequent months. Over the next several years, I did learn new dumbbell exercises and taught myself how to use some of the machines at the gym (by referencing the little helpful stickers on them). However, to my dismay, I wasn't seeing any substantial gains in muscle. I kind of just looked the same even though I was consistently putting in the "work" each week. I had this highly irrational yet visceral fear that if I changed up even the slightest component of my resistance training regimen, all my muscle would be lost. I was paranoid and rigid. Looking back now, I can see how foolish I was, but at the same time, I also want to pat my old self on the back and say, "There, there, Em, it's not your fault." So many of us repeat the same platitude—*if only I knew back then what I know now.*

The thing is that I did know a reasonable amount, and I even got a personal training certificate when I was in college. While the information was useful to a degree, it was more a crash course on anatomy than the training principles that would help me build lean muscle over time.

If you can relate to my sentiments, I want you to know that I really feel for you. When I was training clients in the past, I gave out subpar advice. Okay, it wasn't the worst advice, but it certainly wasn't the best. I was only using the process outlined in my personal training course. Which, by the way, was a weekend-long course—but we'll save my gripe with that for another day. My clients and I made the same mistakes repeatedly, which, in turn, prevented us from making substantial progress toward our body composition goals.

Many people start a program and don't see results even with significant effort and time, so they quit. I honestly don't blame them. There's nothing more discouraging than showing up, doing the work, but seeing little to no progress when it comes to actual changes in body composition.

The information presented in this part of the book is what I wish I knew when I first started my fitness journey in 2008. It would have saved me years of discouragement and frustration. I aim to provide you with the correct information on reaching your fitness goals with training in the simplest and most effective way possible. Akin to nutrition, there's no universal training plan for everyone, and the ones that work best are individualized to suit your commitment levels, lifestyle, and fitness goals. We'll start off with some fundamental definitions to set the stage and then move into how to craft your own plan, the best way to learn new exercises, the role of cardio, tracking workouts, and the importance of sleep. I've also included some sample training plans with exercises that you can follow to a tee or snag what you like from and throw into your plan.

A quick disclaimer: This section is focused more on intermediate trainees who want to build muscle and strength, but beginners can benefit too. Aspiring bodybuilders and powerlifters will want more tailored plans for their respective sports from credible coaches.

TRAINING DEFINITIONS

There's a lot of jargon thrown around in the training world. To avoid throwing out esoteric terminology, let's quickly go over some definitions. If you're unclear, you can revert back to this section or visit the glossary at the back of the book.

Reps: The number of times you perform a single exercise before taking a break.

Sets: The number of *consecutive* reps of a given exercise.

Tempo: The length of time it takes to perform a movement in an exercise. Think of a dance—tempo is like a rhythm. It's the time from your starting position of an exercise, to the top of the movement, then back down to the starting position.

Volume: The amount of work you complete in the gym, usually expressed by the number of sets for a given body part, number of reps per week, and load (how much weight you're lifting).

Progressive overload: If you take anything away from this section, progressive overload is the most vital. Progressive overload means you're doing more work over time to achieve muscle growth (hypertrophy). This could be in the form of increasing the weight, doing more reps, more sets, and/or slowing down the tempo.

Muscle failure: Simply put, muscle failure occurs when you physically cannot perform another repetition. Muscle failure (or getting close to it) is one of the vital ingredients in helping our muscles grow.

Resistance training: Also referred to as weight or strength training; resistance training causes your muscles to contract, which helps you build strength, power, and muscle.

INTRODUCTION TO RESISTANCE TRAINING AND CARDIO

Now that we know a bit of terminology, it's important to understand why resistance training should be part of your fitness plan. Even if you don't really care to put on muscle and you're only looking to lose body fat, I urge you to rethink your stance.

There are innumerable benefits to weight training, which include an increase in your resting metabolism (so you can burn more calories at rest), enhanced performance in your respective sport, improved posture, increased lean muscle mass (which can help with issues as we start to age), and support for bone development.[1]

Traditionally, cardio has been thought of as a fat-burning tool. While cardio does burn more calories in the moment than resistance training does, the muscle mass that we build will really move the needle in our body recomposition efforts. Aside from the aesthetic benefits we can derive, a meta-analysis with over 1,800 participants showed that resistance training can help improve mood and decrease symptoms of depression.[2]

However, I recommend not neglecting cardio, because it offers many benefits as well. A good training plan that includes both resistance training and cardio will make you physically and mentally stronger. Now, let's dive in to how to create your own resistance training plan, uniquely tailored to you and your own personal preferences and fitness goals.

CHAPTER 14

Crafting Your Resistance Training Plan

T he first step in crafting any sort of fitness plan is to try and better understand what you want to achieve. Do you want to develop specific muscle groups? Or do you just want to feel stronger and achieve a more holistically healthy lifestyle? To increase your chances of sticking with a routine long enough to actually see results, you'll want to find a plan that aligns with your commitment levels, training goals, and personal preferences. Let's break these down to get you pondering a bit:

- *Commitment level:* What kind of frequency can you commit to? How many days per week and number of hours per day?

- *Enjoyment:* Do you enjoy weight training or can't stand it? Be honest with yourself.

- *Types of workouts:* Do you prefer a set plan with specific exercises, or do you enjoy variety and mixing things up?

If you're the type of person who doesn't have much time to commit to your workouts and doesn't enjoy training all that much, you'll likely want to focus on an efficient plan that gets you in and out of the gym as quickly as possible and maximizes results. However, if you have more time to commit and get bored easily by repetition, you might want to incorporate more variety in your workouts. If you're not too sure, you can adopt a plan that sounds the most appealing, give it a go, and make individualized tweaks along the way.

Before we get into types of training splits and sample training plans, it's essential to lay out some resistance training best practices to help you achieve your desired results. Reps, sets, and rest between sets are another point of contention in the fitness industry. The recommendations I provide are backed by sound scientific research from some of the best researchers in the field. Keep in mind that these recommendations may go against what you have learned and practice in your training. However, I encourage you to keep an open mind. If you're not getting the results you want with your current plan, try adopting some of these principles. As covered in Part I, unlearning is one of the most difficult but important aspects of making material changes in your physique. By adopting this mindset, you're well on your way.

REPS, SETS, AND REST

How many reps should you complete in a given set, and how many sets should you do of a given exercise? The answer isn't so straightforward. You need to decide your training goals: Are you looking to build muscle (hypertrophy), strength, or muscular endurance? Most of us want to focus on the first one, but it's okay to want all three. It is important to note that the primary goal you choose will affect the number of reps you need to perform per set and the number of sets in a given exercise.

Goal: Muscle Growth (Hypertrophy)

This is the category most of us will fall into. If your goal is to build muscle, you'll need to apply the principles of both progressive overload *and* bringing muscles to technical failure to see growth. The most common rep range for muscle growth is 6–12 reps per set; however, it's still very possible to build muscle doing higher or lower rep ranges. A 2015 study conducted by Brad Schoenfeld and colleagues compared two groups of well-trained men: one group performed 25–35 reps per exercise, and the other performed 8–12 reps per exercise. The findings? The results indicated that both groups' efforts led to hypertrophy.[1] The main point here is that you can see muscle growth across a wide spectrum of rep ranges. However, it may be harder for you to hit muscle (or technical) failure for the higher rep ranges simply because you may tire (from an aerobic standpoint), and I also find that doing too many exercises with high reps can get boring—I'm more likely to stop the set before hitting technical failure.

I encourage you, therefore, to stay in the lower rep range (6–15 reps), with a focus on hitting muscle failure (when you physically cannot perform one more rep) within the last *set* of each given exercise. Two to three sets per exercise is generally a good rule of thumb to follow. For hypertrophy, the ideal rest time is one to two minutes between sets. Short rest periods such as these have been proven to increase blood flow, which helps protein get to the muscles at a more rapid rate.

Goal: Build Strength

If your goal is to build strength, the recommended rep range drops quite a bit. Powerlifters would fit nicely into this category, but it is also for individuals who just want to get stronger and lift more. The suggested rep range for strength training is one to five reps per set, while lifting the heaviest weight out of all the other training methods. Generally, two to five sets per *exercise* is a good rule of thumb to follow to build strength. From a strength perspective, that includes lower reps, and most studies recommend a rest period of three to five minutes between sets.

Goal: Build Endurance

When your body performs for longer periods of time, it uses slow-twitch muscle fibers, providing you with the endurance to last longer during exercise. To train for endurance, you need to lower the weight a bit and focus on lifting lighter loads (15 reps or more), with less rest between sets. By incorporating lighter weight and more reps, your body will be able to better utilize oxygen and give you that added boost of energy. If you're a runner, working on endurance can help you sustain harder periods of activity for longer. Another added benefit of building endurance is that you will burn more calories while boosting your metabolism. The number of sets should also be higher and typically ranges from two to four sets to two to six sets per exercise. To increase stamina, it's recommended to take 45 seconds to two minutes between sets. Even if your goal is to build muscle, strength, and power, working on endurance can be a great primer (as a warm-up) or a finisher, which can provide some added benefits similar to those of cardio.

A Hybrid Approach: The Powerbuilding Workout Program

While I have defined hypertrophy, strength, and endurance as separate goals, a good progressive resistance training plan combines all three. For body recomposition, personal trainer and founder of the popular YouTube channel Anabolic Aliens, Mike Rosa recommends following a "progressive powerbuilding workout plan." He defines powerbuilding as "a type of training that mixes powerlifting and bodybuilding techniques." Rosa's program incorporates both strength (1–5 reps to failure) and hypertrophy (6–12 reps to failure). Rosa points out that there's a correlation between strength and gaining muscle. He writes, "The stronger you are, the more muscle building potential you have."[2] For this reason, Rosa recommends starting the workout with one to two strength-focused, compound exercises (more on this soon) and then focusing the remainder of the workout on the rep range for muscle growth. You could throw in some endurance work at the beginning of the workout (primer) or at the end (finisher).

VOLUME AND FREQUENCY

In addition to the principle of progressive overload, training volume is also a main driver of muscle growth. Volume refers to the number of sets, reps, and load (the weight you lift) in a given week. The general consensus is that 10–30 sets per body part per week, with some outliers, is optimal. However, it's worth noting that some studies conducted on trained athletes upped the volume to 30–45 sets per week and found that the participants saw significant growth.[3] Most beginners, however, typically aim for around 10 sets per week, while intermediate and advanced athletes aim for closer to 20 sets per week.

Training frequency refers to the number of times you work a muscle in a given week. So, if you're a beginner, you could do 5 sets of back exercises and repeat the session sometime during the week, or you could do 10 sets of back exercises in a single session. If you're at an intermediate level or more advanced, you could up that to 10 sets or more. But *does frequency matter in relation to maximizing hypertrophy (muscle growth)?*

A 2016 study by Schoenfeld and colleagues looked at training frequency from one to three days per week while keeping volume the same across all groups. The study concluded that training at least twice per week promoted more muscle growth than training each muscle group once per week.[4] However, more recent studies show that hypertrophy is driven more by volume than frequency.

Schoenfeld and colleagues published a more recent systemic review and meta-analysis that looked at 25 studies that met certain inclusion criteria. The researchers concluded that "there is strong evidence that resistance training frequency does not significantly or meaningfully impact muscle hypertrophy when volume is equated."[5]

So when crafting your plan to maximize muscle gain, it doesn't seem to matter how many times per week you work out specific muscle groups, as long as volume is matched. However, many of us will likely benefit by distributing the volume throughout multiple days (instead of a single day), which can aid in our recovery efforts.

As for volume, it's best to determine how many sets you should do by setting a range and tracking your progress. You'll also want to get an idea on how your body is feeling from a recovery standpoint. If you're really sore and find that recovery times are long, you might want to bring volume down, which will reduce your risk of injury. If you're at a stall or plateau, however, you might want to increase your weekly volume.

A good question to ask yourself is: Am I seeing muscle growth and getting stronger each week? If your answer is yes, then the set volume you're doing is probably okay. If you plateau and your muscle gain is more incremental, you might want to subsequently increase the volume. However, there is a point where you'll max out, so listen to your body. If you're in pain or recovery time between sessions is increasingly longer, it's a clear indication that you're overtraining and might want to scale it back.

TRAINING INTENSITY

Training intensity is how hard you're working in the gym and an important stress variable in building muscular adaptations. In the 1970s, the Borg Scale, developed by Swedish physiologist and researcher Gunnar Borg, was the most widely used method to measure aerobic exercise intensity based on a person's self-perceived efforts. The ratings ranged from 6 to 20, based on a combination of heart rate, breathlessness, and fatigue. The lowest end of the scale (6) equated to minimal to no effort, and the highest side (20) was considered an all-out effort. The rating was supposed to correlate with heart rate by adding a zero to the end of each number. The lower end of a normal resting heart rate for adults is 60 (hence the seeming randomness of starting at 6).

So, say you're doing sprints, and you feel like you're working at an 18, your heart rate should measure close to 180 beats per minute (bpm). The moderate level would fall into the 12–14 range (120–140 bpm). A newer, modified version of the Borg Scale measures perceived exertion out of 10. Of course, there are some drawbacks with this method because heart rate can vary from individual to individual.[6]

A more recent and widely used rate of perceived exertion (RPE) scale rates perceived effort on a scale from 1–10 and isn't based on heart rate. Since Borg was traditionally used for aerobic exercise only, the modified scale has been adopted by strength trainees as well. The scale can be summarized for aerobic activity in the following table.

Rate of perceived exertion	Intensity, or "zones"	Examples
RPE 1–2	Easy/light	Walking
RPE 3–4	Moderate	Light jog, steady-state cardio
RPE 5–6	Hard	Tempo run
RPE 7–8	Very hard	VO2 max training
RPE 9–10	Max/all-out effort	Sprinting/race pace

To quantify their efforts in the gym, weight lifters have adapted the RPE scale to indicate the number of *reps to failure* or the number of *reps in reserve*.[7] The scale quantifies weight-lifting efforts in the gym using a numerical approach to determine how many more reps can be done before hitting muscle failure in a given set. A RPE rating of 10 would mean you gave your lift an all-out effort, reaching technical muscle failure. An 8 or 9 is still extremely difficult; you pushed very hard but didn't quite hit your max (you feel like you could have gotten another one or two reps in before reaching failure). Reps in reserve, or RIR, is the inverse of RPE (so a rating of 1 means you have one rep left in the tank before muscle failure, a RIR of 2 means two reps, and so on and so forth). For the sake of simplicity when crafting your plan, I suggest using RIR for weight lifting to avoid confusion with the traditional RPE scale.

Like any subjective scales, there are, of course, downsides. The big issue with the RIR scale is that it's too subjective, and research has shown that most people are poor at evaluating their own perceived effort in the gym.[8] In fact, we typically overestimate our perceived efforts by thinking we're working harder than we really are. Since training intensity is one of the most important variables in muscle adaptation, not working hard enough when we think we are can really stunt our progress. This is more common with beginner and novice trainees who are still learning what muscle "failure" feels like. As you progress and get more advanced, you'll get better at estimating when you're hitting muscle failure or getting close. It's an essential skill that you can develop over time.

So how hard should you push in your workout? If there's any heated debate among the fitness and scientific community, it's this one. The intensity of your training depends on your goals, your experience level, and how fast you can recover between workouts. The consensus is that you shouldn't be training at an RIR of 0–1 every single session but, rather, should be breaking out your training into cycles.

TRAINING PHASES FOR BUILDING MUSCLE

When crafting your training plan, you'll want to view it in cycles or phases (similar to the bulking and cutting protocols I cover in Part II). Training phases are a way to gradually build your fitness level over time and can be used both in aerobic and strength training.[9] A phase will allow you to incorporate harder workouts, which gives your body enough stressors to build muscle while also allowing for ample recovery—a key building block in muscular adaptations. Let's review the three training phases, or what is known as *periodization*:

1. *Macrocycle:* This phase is what you would consider a full season, so whatever that looks like for you. For example, a macrocycle could be six months or even a year. It gives you a holistic view of your training plan.

2. *Mesocycle:* This phase is a training block of time within a particular season (typically three to four weeks, but it can also be four to six weeks or longer).

3. *Microcycle:* This phase is an amount of time within a mesocycle (typically a week or so).

The goal with periodization is to accumulate lean muscle at a safe but steady rate while minimizing the risk of injury. This doesn't apply to just weight lifters in the gym; many elite athletes will align their training with periodization for competition to maximize their performance. The phase is not a set-in-stone plan; rather, it can be individualized by taking into account your starting point and experience with weight lifting.

There are a few different models of periodization, but two popular ones are the *linear progression (LP) model* and the *undulating model (DUP)*.[10] In the linear progression model, you make steady progression over time—each training session you add more volume (reps/sets/weight) and train at high intensity during each session. This model is most commonly recommended for novices/beginners. But as you progress and become more advanced, pushing to your limits during each workout is a bit riskier and can lead to injury and slower recovery time. The undulating model looks at weekly or daily workouts and mixes in some easier sessions with harder ones. This model allows you to train with enough intensity in a given block of time to cause muscle failure, while allowing your body ample recovery time in between blocks.

Some undulating models can last between four and six weeks, and after each mesocycle, you should gain strength and progressively add more volume each week—until, of course, you hit a bit of a ceiling with your body composition. The following sections provide an example of what a four-week mesocycle would look like.

Week 1–3

Start training at an RIR of 3 (7 RPE) with lower volume so that you feel like you've had a good workout and perhaps get a bit sore but not sore enough to hinder your next workout. Stick with a similar intensity (maintaining a 3, maybe a 4 RIR) each week, but slowly add more volume (sets/reps/weight) over the progression of the next two weeks. Keep in mind that you want to be recovered enough to work out at a similar intensity without feeling so sore that it hinders your gains. This is the accumulation phase, in which you'll be building up to your maximum intensity and priming your body to really push in week 4. You'll be focusing on good form and technique, so when you really stack on the weight in the last week, you'll be better equipped to handle the load.

Week 4

In week 4 you'll try pushing at your maximum intensity. That is, for the *last set* of each exercise, you're going to want to achieve muscle failure or hit a 0–1 RIR (90–100% in one-repetition maximum/1RM, or maximum amount of weight an individual can lift in a single repetition with proper form). At this point, you're going to feel very fatigued after your workouts. Adding any more volume or intensity will reverse any effects because muscle adaptations will take a nosedive, which can lead to overtraining and injury. You'll then want to repeat the cycle, starting back at week 1, bringing down the training volume a bit, and keeping your RIR to around 3 or so.

A Few Rules of Thumb

Personal trainer, physique coach, and researcher Dr. Eric Helms suggests that you need to have an RIR of at least a 4 or higher (RPE > 6) most of the time and be "reasonably close to failure" to see adaptations.[11] Helms also suggests that we should be mostly in the RIR range of 1–3 or RPE range of 7–9 to induce hypertrophy. RIR is highly individualized and a subjective measure of how you're feeling when you leave the gym. "It has to feel like a high level of tension," says Helms.[12] Are you feeling fatigued or fully wiped? A rule of thumb Helms suggests is that muscles should be fully recovered within three days of a training session. If they aren't, your volume or intensity is too high, and you should scale it back. If in any way during the accumulation phase you feel your workouts are too easy, you may want to up the volume.

TRAINING SPLITS

A training split is a resistance training program that breaks out training sessions by body parts or muscle groups. Before we dive into some examples of popular splits, the following is a breakdown of the major muscle groups and a few of the associated muscles:

Muscle group	Major muscles
Chest	Upper, middle, lower pecs
Arms	Biceps Triceps Forearms
Back	Latissimus dorsi (lats) Traps Rhomboids
Shoulders	Front, side, and rear deltoids Rotator cuffs
Legs	Quadriceps Hamstrings Glutes
Calves	Calves
Abdominals	Rectus abdominus Obliques

Full Body

Full-body workouts are exactly how they sound; instead of breaking out your strength sessions by particular body parts, you'll be working out your entire body. Full body workouts are simple, straightforward, and if you include compound exercises (more on this soon), you don't need to spend endless hours in the gym. I typically recommended full-body splits to beginners, but this type of workout is also a good option for anyone who doesn't want to spend too much time at the gym. For full body, a three- to four-day split is ideal, but you can also choose just two days. Full body is great because you can easily schedule in rest days and take weekends off if you so desire. The following are a few examples of what the full-body split would look like:

TWO DAYS

Monday: Full body
Tuesday: Rest
Wednesday: Rest
Thursday: Full body

THREE DAYS

Monday: Full body
Tuesday: Rest
Wednesday: Full body
Thursday: Rest
Friday: Full body

FOUR DAYS

Monday: Full body
Tuesday: Rest
Wednesday: Full body
Thursday: Rest
Friday: Full body
Saturday: Rest
Sunday: Full body

Upper/Lower Body

Upper- and lower-body splits are the most common and are considered to be one of the most optimal of the splits to achieve muscle growth. These are great for anyone on a more intermediate level but also for beginners. On the upper-body days, you'll work your chest, shoulders, biceps, and triceps. On the lower-body days, you'll work quads, calves, hamstrings, and glutes. You can also choose to do core in either the lower- or upper-body days. The most common split is four days, in which you'll work each section of the body twice. For example, an upper/lower-body split would look like the following:

Monday: Upper body
Tuesday: Lower body
Wednesday: Rest
Thursday: Upper body
Friday: Lower body

Push/Pull or Body Part Split

With the push/pull split, you're scheduling your training by combining multiple body parts in a single day. It's a great way to increase strength and better develop specific body parts. *Push* means that the weight is being pushed away from your body, while *pull* means weight is being pulled toward your body. A push split includes chest, shoulders, triceps, quads, and calves. A pull split includes traps, back, biceps, and hamstrings. Similar to the upper/lower-body split, you can include core exercises in either the push or pull days. The push/pull splits are typically more for advanced trainees. It is the split that I currently use and the one where I finally started to see my palpable changes in my physique. For example, a push/pull split would look like the following:

Monday: Push
Tuesday: Pull
Wednesday: Rest
Thursday: Push
Friday: Pull

The Hybrid Approach

Depending on your own personal goals, you might want to consider combining splits. For example, I occasionally use an upper-body push/pull split and the lower-body split. I also like to break out my shoulders into their own day because aesthetically, I like the look of well-defined shoulders and my rear delts are also a weaker point of mine. I also don't care too much about developing my chest or triceps. Here's a quick example of my current training plan:

Monday: Upper-body pull (biceps, back, traps)
Tuesday: Lower body (legs, core)
Wednesday: Upper-body push
Thursday: Lower body
Friday: Upper-body pull
Saturday: Shoulders
Sunday: Rest

Which Split Should You Choose?

For beginners and for those who want efficiency in their workouts, I'd recommend either the full body or upper/lower split. If you're at an intermediary level or more advanced, you can choose the push/pull or upper/lower split, as these are usually the most optimal to develop improvements in strength and hypertrophy. I encourage you to try different splits and see what works for you! I like to switch mine up every so often because I enjoy variety, and as you can see from my previous example, I want to develop weaker areas more than others. I therefore tailor my plan to fit my individualized goals, and I encourage you to do the same.

TYPES OF EXERCISES

Now that we have a base level understanding of training terminology and the types of training splits we can choose from, let's figure out what type of exercises to include in your plan.

Exercises can be broken out into two types: *compound* and *isolation*. Let's go through what each type is to help you determine which is the most optimal for you.

Compound Exercises

Compound exercises are exercises that work more than one body part at a time. These exercises will give you the most bang for your workout buck.

Compound exercises pros

- Time-efficient
- Lead to better gains in muscle growth
- Easier to track progress
- Improve performance, strength, and power
- Help improve stability and balance
- Help burn more calories in your workout
- Can elicit a greater metabolic response

Compound exercises cons

- Can be boring and repetitious, since there are only so many compound movements you can do
- Some compound movements are difficult to perform (e.g., dead lifts)
- Improper form can lead to injury

Examples of compound exercises

Exercise	Target muscle groups
Dead lifts	Hamstrings, glutes, lower and mid-back, lats, and forearms
Squats	Quads, hamstrings, abs, calves, and glutes
Chest press	Delts, chest, and triceps
Barbell row	Lats and biceps
Overhead barbell press	Chest, shoulders, arms, and upper back

Isolation Exercises

Isolation exercises work a certain body part or area to focus on a specific muscle or joint.

Isolation exercises pros

- Help you improve weak areas or muscle imbalances

- Provide more muscle growth in specific areas

- Performed with lighter weight, resulting in a lower likelihood of injury

- Are typically easier to perform than compound

- Help regain strength (if you're sustaining or have sustained an injury), without further damaging muscle

Isolation exercises cons

- Require more time in the gym

- Burn fewer calories than compound exercises

Examples of isolation exercises

Exercise	Target muscle groups
Leg curl	Hamstrings
Bicep curl	Biceps
Lateral raises	Side deltoid
Tricep extensions	Triceps

Which Type of Exercise to Choose?

If your goal is to build muscle or gain strength (performance-related), compound movements should make up the bulk of your routine. However, it's important to prioritize the exercises that work the largest muscle groups first then move on to the isolation exercises. Not only are compound exercises the most efficient, but they allow us to lift more (stimulating hypertrophy), making it easier to achieve and track week-over-week progression.

Some trainers recommend only compound exercises and minimize isolation (if isolation exercises are even included at all). Without isolation exercises, however, we may be missing out on more muscle growth in specific areas that compound movements don't emphasize (e.g., triceps). In my opinion, incorporating only compound exercises can be straight-up boring.

Isolation also allows you to add more *volume* to existing body parts. In sum, compound exercises should be primary and isolation secondary. To which degree you want to include each is based on your own preferences. You could probably get away with just doing compound, but it's good to have a mix (and also variety). I personally enjoy doing isolation exercises more than compound and include quite a few in my routine.

The type of exercises you choose depends on your time commitment in the gym, and whether you like structure and routine or prefer more variety and mixing things up more often. Enjoyment is another big one—I hate doing squats, for example, so I don't do them. Just because an exercise is effective in hitting multiple muscle groups and optimizing your time doesn't mean it will be enjoyable for you. Remember that our goal is sustainability; we want to land on not only a routine that garners results but also one that we can stick with over the long haul.

BUILDING MUSCLE: FREE WEIGHTS VERSUS MACHINES

When it comes to building muscle, both free weights and machines can get the job done. Each have their pros and cons, but a well-built training plan will include both (if you have access to them).

Free Weights

Free weights require more control than machines do. To minimize the chance of injury, it's important to learn good form while performing exercises with free weights. Akin to compound exercises, the big pro with free weights is that they typically work more muscle groups than machines do (with the exception of a few). Most compound exercises are performed with free weights or barbells. For example, if you are doing an overhead shoulder press, you are working not only your shoulders but also your chest, triceps, traps, and pecs—plus you're engaging your core. More advanced lifters typically structure their plans to include a majority of free weights and use machines as an "accessory" to isolate certain muscle groups or work on weaker areas.

Machines

If you're a beginner, machines are a great starting point because they can teach you proper form and reduce the risk of injury. If you're seeking efficiency in the gym, free weights may be the way to go, but there are several machines that can hit multiple major muscle groups. My favorites are the seated row and the lateral pull-down machine. The biggest downside from using the machines, however, is that they aren't super customizable. When doing a seated leg extension, for instance, I can't seem to adjust the settings to get the machine placed just right on my shins; it's either too close to my ankles or too far up my leg. Some machines are better at adjusting than others, but depending on your build, some machines may be hard to configure to do the exercises comfortably.

The scientific community has long debated whether free weights or machines are better. However, as long as training volume is consistent across groups, research has shown that training with either free weights or machines has similar effects on building strength and muscle mass.[13]

Assuming you've done some resistance training, I'd recommend focusing primarily on free weights and using machines to target underdeveloped areas or to isolate areas your free weights may miss. Once again, the most important training variables are progressive overload (which can be done with both free weights and machines) and getting in those hard sets to reach muscle failure.

LEARNING NEW EXERCISES AND FORM

While I could include diagrams of exercises and explanations of each movement, I don't think that's the optimal way to learn new exercises and practice proper form. Working with a trainer to show you how to properly perform exercises is the most optimal, albeit most expensive option. However, hiring a trainer, even for just a few sessions, could be a worthwhile investment.

If you're like me, however, and like to figure out things for yourself, then finding good resources on learning various exercises is a must. For isolation exercises and adding more variety to your workouts, I always recommend one resource: Mike Rosa's YouTube channel, Anabolic Aliens. Rosa's workouts have been an invaluable resource for me in building my strength and changing my physique. In my opinion, it is, hands down, the best YouTube channel to learn new exercises. Rosa's workouts are highly targeted to specific muscle groups and body parts. He's not only found preexisting exercises but also designed many himself. When building out your training split, try doing a few of these workouts, and as you repeat them week over week, you'll naturally start learning the exercises and proper form.

Many of Rosa's videos are focused on endurance (getting as many reps as possible in a specific time frame), but once you learn the exercises, you can increase the weight and incorporate them into your regular routine. For me, I prefer to do two to three videos three times a week before I begin lifting any heavier. You can also use these videos as a primer, finisher, or piece together a few of the videos for your entire workout.

REST AND RECOVERY

Not giving your body adequate rest between training sessions is one of the biggest mistakes you can make in your training. In *Peak Performance*, Brad Stulberg and Steve Magness deduce the following growth equation: Stress + Rest = Growth. If you lean too much on the former, you risk burnout and injury. If you lean too much on the latter, you impede progress, or plateau, and get stuck in complacency.

Overtraining can be a dangerous game. It can not only lead to injury but also adversely affect your progress. You can even lose strength from training too much. Overtraining syndrome can cause inflammation to your nervous system and cause chronic fatigue, low moods, burnout, bad sleep, and even depression.[14]

Scheduling rest days and deloading periods, where you scale back on your training volume and intensity, are critical in helping you make progress. Furthermore, when you train, your body creates micro tears in your muscles. Your muscles don't actually grow when you're training (even though the inflammation can give you that "pump" or "swole" appearance). The muscle growth is in your workout's aftermath—when you're in a resting state and your body works to repair and build new muscle tissue.

How much rest do you need between training sessions then? This depends on the individual, but rest days should be scheduled for at least one day between training sessions, possibly two days (for specific muscle groups—for example, you don't want to work out the same muscle groups back-to-back). If you're feeling abnormally sore and having a difficult time recovering, you may be doing too much volume in the gym and might want to scale that back a bit. It's okay to be a bit sore, but if you're in physical pain, then that's a strong indication that you need more rest. Symptoms of burnout, fatigue, or bad sleep may also be signals that it's time to scale back. The last variable is performance related. Plateaus will happen—it's an inevitable part of your training. If you feel like your strength isn't increasing for some time, you may be either not working hard enough, or working too hard and not giving your body adequate rest.

Deloading Periods

When training for a marathon, runners build up their mileage over the course of months and then, just weeks before the big race, they get in a last long run before tapering their training.

This tapering or "deloading" is where you reduce your training loads and intensity or take a full stop on training for a specific period of time.

When it comes to resistance training, a common piece of advice dished out by coaches/trainers is to train for three weeks and take one week off or significantly reduce your training in that last week. Other common advice is to train for eight weeks and take one week off. But taking a full week off training is more a myth than anything.

Personal trainer and fitness expert Menno Henselmans recommends using "reactive deloads" rather than taking a full week off. This means listening to your body, watching progress, and giving yourself rest periods when you start to see performance decline. Rather than proactively planning rest periods, Menno recommends scheduling the time based on your individual needs. Take the deload period on specific muscle groups rather than from your full-body workouts.[15]

Many people (including myself) have been training for years and don't ever take full weeks off their training. I do, however, scale back on the intensity of my sessions or schedule an additional rest day if needed. If you're experiencing any overtraining symptoms, it's a good idea to take extra rest or scale back on the training volume (one-third to two-thirds of what you normally do) and lower the intensity (at about a 6–7 RPE or a 3–4 RIR).

Types of Recovery—Passive versus Active

When most people think of rest or recovery, their minds go to their bodies not doing anything at all. This type of recovery is coined as "passive" and involves sitting, sleeping, or barely performing any physical movement. The less ubiquitous form is "active recovery," and this involves performing some light, non-strenuous strength exercises or low-intensity cardio in the day or day(s) following a high-intensity workout.

Passive recovery is a good route to take if you're recovering from an injury, illness, or mental/physical fatigue and exhaustion. Allowing your body to rest completely can be beneficial for a speedy recovery.

However, for most workouts, active recovery is usually the best way to go. After a hard training session, even some stretching and light walking is better than sitting on your bum on the couch all day. Active recovery can help increase blood flow, reduce lactic acid in our muscles (from strenuous training), and help with flexibility and mobility.

A 2010 study looked at 25 trained swimmers and the effects of active and passive recovery on performance in a two-day period. On the first day, the swimmers performed active recovery where they performed regeneration exercises, and on the second day, the swimmers rested (passive). Immediately following their training, blood lactate levels rose to 78%. On the active rest days, the lactate dissipated at a faster rate than on passive rest days. The study concluded that active rest days, that include light exercise, can help improve athletic performance more than passive rest.[16]

So not only can active rest help us recover faster, but it can also potentially increase performance. Numerous studies have outlined the benefits of active recovery in endurance athletes. I always bring down my mileage and do some low-intensity cardio the day after a hard training session. Especially when delayed-muscle onset (as the name implies: delayed muscle soreness) is at its strongest, I find some active recovery always makes me feel more limber and ready to get back at it the next day.

Nutrition on Rest Days

Just because you're not doing as much activity on rest days doesn't mean you need to drop your calories. Keep calories the same as your plan entails. Some people on a deficit will even bring their bodies back up to maintenance to give their body adequate nutrition to recover. Listen to your body and don't try to deprive yourself or feel guilty because you're eating at the same caloric intake as you are on training days. Since muscle protein synthesis can typically be elevated for up to 48 hours after a hard resistance-training session, it's vital that we're still feeding out bodies with optimal protein. Continue to track your protein intake and try to hit your daily targets.

TRAINING DIFFERENCES IN WOMEN

While I tried to write this book and provide general recommendations for all genders, I would be remiss without mentioning some biological differences in how cis men and cis women train. This section is specifically for women and how you can tweak your plan slightly (emphasis on *slightly*) to optimize your results. Let's start by addressing the following common myths.

Myth 1: Lifting Weights Will Make You "Bulky"

One of the most annoying myths and repeated phrases I hear from other cis women is that they think lifting weights will make them "bulky." Trust me, you won't get bulky. Unless you're following a rigorous progressive training plan and purposely eating in a caloric surplus for a long time, you're not going to get big. As a cis woman, putting on muscle has taken an exuberant amount of effort, consistency, and meticulous planning. My training has been years in the making and I still don't have that "she-hulk" look.

The only thing lifting weights will do is improve your body composition, achieve a toned look, help you trim down on the fat, increase your confidence, improve your athletic performance, and make you an all-around healthier person. Now that I've gotten that out of the way, let's move on.

Myth 2: Women Have a Genetic Disadvantage

On the inverse side, there's a myth that because women don't have as much testosterone than men, then we won't be able to put on that much lean muscle mass without the use of some sort of drug. I've personally been asked on several occasions if I take some form of steroid—the answer is a hard *no*.

First off, testosterone is not a determinant of muscle growth in women; other, more complex hormones and anabolic responses are at play. Further, women have just as much potential to naturally build muscle as men do. Menno Henselmans wrote a fantastic article in which he points to several scientific studies that examine the potential of strength building in women. Henselmans writes, "The only difference is the starting point. Men start off with more muscle mass and more strength, but the relative increase in muscle size is the same between men and women."[17]

A 2001 study looked at how age and gender affected muscle growth from strength training efforts. The study took four groups—young men (ages 20–30), young women (ages 20–30), older men (ages 65–75), and older women (ages 65–75)—and put them through a six-month strength training program. At the end of the six-month period, the study concluded that "neither age nor gender affects muscle volume response to whole body strength training."[18]

So it's clear that women do have the potential to gain strength and muscle. We may even be at more of an advantage to gain muscle because of our naturally higher body fat percentages and the positive roles estrogen can play. Another myth is that estrogen is the enemy when it comes to building muscle. However, that is simply not true. In fact, estrogen is our friend. This hormone can help prevent muscle loss (has anti-catabolic properties), can aid in muscle repair, and even increase metabolism.[19]

So now that we know that women have the potential to build muscle and that resistance training won't make us bulky, let's dive in to some of the tweaks you may want to make to your training. First, let me emphasize the word *tweak*. Women do not need an entirely different training plan, but you can make some variations to capitalize on your gender's strengths.

Training Volume and Women

Women have more slow-twitch muscle fibers (type-I and -IIA) than men do, which means that women don't tire as quickly from our workouts.[20] We can, therefore, typically perform more reps per set than men can, and women also don't need as much rest between sets as men do.[21] Women can typically perform more reps at a lower tempo or "slower cadence" than men, which can help us maximize muscle size.[22]

Estrogen's role in recovery means that women can handle more volume (hard sets per muscle group) in a given week. In addition, women are able to perform more sets with more intensity, recover faster, and with less risk of injury.

Now that we know that training volume correlates strongest with muscle adaptations, we have a lot of potential to increase strength. Women can typically go higher than men in a given week. Volume-wise I normally perform 30 sets or more per muscle group per week, which is much more than the more common recommendation of 10–20 sets.

Explosive Movements and Women

Explosive movements (for example, sprinting and powerlifting), however, are where women are left with a bit of a disadvantage. Men typically perform better at explosive movements, so by training with less explosive movements, women can better take advantage of their genetic strengths and muscle adaptations in the gym.[23] It usually takes women longer to recover from a high-intensity interval training (HIIT) treadmill workout or dynamic exercises (such as jumping squats).

Because of our slow-twitch muscle fibers, women are better suited to endurance exercise, which includes low-intensity, steady-state cardio or endurance events. Women also do particularly well in running ultramarathons.

However, just because women don't do as well as men in explosive exercises doesn't mean we shouldn't include them in our workouts (I discuss this more in the next chapter). I only incorporate these type of workouts one to two times per week max because my recovery time is quite long. So just note that genetically we may take longer to recover from the explosive types of workouts. However, if you enjoy these exercises, then definitely include them!

Key Takeaways for Women

- Women have as much potential to gain strength and muscle size than men *without the use of drugs.*

- Estrogen helps aid in women's muscle recovery and repair and plays a role in metabolic processes, which allows women to recover faster during workouts.

- Women typically benefit from slower tempos when lifting.

- Women can handle more training volume (sets, reps) per week than men because of our speed and recovery.

- Research shows that women *typically* perform better at lower-intensity cardio and less explosive movements. However, we should still include explosive movements in our training.

SAMPLE TRAINING PLAN

I end this chapter with a sample training plan to give you a starting point, or to jump-start setting up your own plan. The following is an example of my current training plan. My friend Mike Rosa graciously put together some sample training plans for you based on each of the aforementioned splits (located in the Resources section at the back of the book).

Hybrid Plan: Upper Push/Pull and Lower-Body Split

Monday: Upper-body pull workout (biceps, back, traps)

Muscle growth (3–4 sets, 6–12 reps per set)
Volume: 18–24 sets total

EXERCISES:

Alternating bicep curls
Wide row
Barbell drag curl
Seated row
Back shrugs
Barbell shrugs

Tuesday: Lower body and core

Muscle growth (3–4 sets, 6–12 reps per set)
Volume: 27–36 sets total

CORE EXERCISES:

Lying leg raises
Bicycle crunches
Russian twists
Side bends
Dumbbell snatches
Volume: 15–20 sets total

LEG EXERCISES:

Weighted calf raises
Leg press
Seated leg extension
Goblet squats
Volume: 12–16 sets total

Wednesday: Upper-body push workout (shoulders, chest, triceps)

Muscle growth (3–4 sets, 6–12 reps per set)
Volume: 45–60 sets total

SHOULDERS:	CHEST:	TRICEPS:
Arnold press	Standing fly	Bench dips
Front raise	Squeeze press	Rope triceps pushdown
Bent-over reverse fly	Svend press	Overhead
Lateral raise	Reverse press	triceps extension
Upright row	Standing chest press	Skull crushers
		Bent-over triceps extensions

Thursday: Core

3–4 sets, 8–15 reps*
Volume: 15–20 sets total

EXERCISES:

Side bends (with 50-lb. weights)
Flutter kicks
C-sit hold
Toe touches
Reverse crunches

*I personally go a bit higher with reps on core exercises

Friday: Upper-body pull workout (biceps, back, traps)

Muscle growth (3–4 sets, 8–12 reps per set)
Volume: 21–28 sets total

EXERCISES:

Dumbbell straight curl
Dumbbell pullover
Alternating dumbbell curls
Front shrugs
Standing cable curl
Bent-over row
Overhead shrugs

Saturday: Shoulders

Muscle growth (3 sets, 8–12 reps per set)
Volume: 18 sets total

EXERCISES:

Alternating dumbbell front raise
Bent-over reverse fly
Seated lateral raise
Y rear delt fly
Bent-arm lateral raise

Strength (3 sets, 4–6 reps per set)

EXERCISE:

Seated shoulder press

CHAPTER 15

The Role of Cardio

Cardiovascular exercise, or "cardio" for short, is a form of aerobic exercise that engages your respiratory system and heart—strengthening both. Cardio has been traditionally viewed as a weight-loss tool but more recently has been a point of contention among the fitness community. Over the years, I've seen the same questions pop up frequently: *How much cardio should I include in my workouts? What type of cardio is best? Will cardio "kill my gains" (impede muscle growth)? Do I even need cardio to hit my body recomp goals?*

In this chapter, we cover all these questions while also providing you with the tools to determine how much cardio you should include in your plan. Some trainers recommend little to no cardio in their workouts (as it could possibly impede muscle growth), while others recommend much more cardio, and some are more in the middle. As a gal who runs every day, I obviously have a biased opinion about cardio—I love it. But I'm aware that others chant the mantra "Cardio is hardio"—they hate it. Regardless of whether you love it or hate it, I think cardio (if done right) plays a vital role not only in helping you expedite fat loss but also in supporting your overall physical and mental well-being.

BENEFITS OF CARDIO

When most people think of losing weight or fat, they envision themselves slaving away on a cardio machine such as a treadmill, elliptical, or stationary bike—wiping off their hard-earned sweat moustaches with their little gym towel. While cardio does help expedite fat loss, there are also many other understated benefits of aerobic exercise that affect both your physical and mental health:

- *Overall health:* In short, cardio is really good for you, as it can reduce blood pressure, increase insulin sensitivity, lower the risk of cardiovascular disease, strengthen your immune system, and is a great workout for our hearts.[1]

- *Recovery and performance:* Low-intensity cardio (active recovery) following a tough training session can help our bodies clear blood lactate, improve athletic performance, and help us recover faster from our workouts.

- *Fat loss:* Cardio can help us burn more calories, which helps us expedite fat loss. In short, if we include some cardio in our training plans, we can eat more!

- *Mood booster:* We've all experienced that quotidian "runner's high," which is that surge of energy and good mood you feel following a cardio session.

- *Effects on the brain:* New research has emerged on the effects aerobic exercise has on the brain. In his book *Spark: The Revolutionary New Science of Exercise and the Brain*, John D. Ratey writes:

  > Exercise provides an unparalleled stimulus, creating an environment in which the brain is ready, willing, and able to learn. Aerobic activity has a dramatic effect on adaptation, regulating systems that might be out of balance and optimizing those that are not—it's an indispensable tool for anyone who wants to reach [their] full potential.[2]

- A bout of cardio can help us bring more focus to our work, increase our ability to learn at a cellular level, and help us better regulate hormones in the brain.

- Cardio's benefits are immense, and aerobic exercise reaches far beyond the "fat loss" side of things. You can see now why I'm biased toward cardio and why I think that no matter what your goals are, you should include aerobic exercise in your training to some extent.

CHALLENGES WITH CARDIO

I think some people starting out with cardio are deterred because it *feels* difficult if you haven't built up your stamina. But even if you're not very good at cardio and struggle at first, if you stick with it, slowly you will become better. Hopefully, it won't feel so much like hell and torture for you. It's just those initial stages that you really need to push through. As you continue to improve, you'll feel a surge of motivation to keep progressing and even doing higher intensities for longer durations.

I started running back in 2008 for the sole reason to lose weight. However, over time, the activity has provided much more meaning to me. I would say running is now an ardent love. As the years progress, I discover new and amazing benefits to running—it's my secret weapon to combat stress, clear my head, and subdue my stream of self-deprecating thoughts.

Mindset is important here. If you frame cardio as a fat-loss tool only, you're likely not going to enjoy it very much. It will feel more akin to torture than enjoyment. When I go into my cardio session thinking "calories in versus calories out," I find it highly demotivating and end up suffering through my workout. If, on the other hand, I use my workout as *me time*—to think through difficult problems, brainstorm ideas, enjoy the solitude of the trails, or plug in to a good audiobook, I'm more present—my running becomes much more enjoyable. Cardio becomes autotelic; I'm motivated by the act of simply running and not by the attainment of an external reward.

I suggest testing out other mental frameworks to enjoy cardio more (as discussed in Part I). Jot down or make a mental note of the other benefits you experience after a good workout and remember those for your next session. Remember, the intrinsic and deeper meaning we assign to our training is a key to sustainability.

CONTROVERSIES SURROUNDING CARDIO

Many coaches or trainers recommend keeping cardio to a minimum or shying away from it altogether if you want to *maximize* muscle growth. Said trainers claim cardio can "kill your gains" and impede hypertrophy. Some others go so far as to say that long-distance runners won't be able to gain much muscle mass at all. While there is some merit in these statements, the actual extent to which aerobic exercise impedes your muscle growth depends on the type of cardio you're doing, as well as the frequency and the body part you're trying to develop. It can't be boiled down to a one-word answer.

The long-held belief that combining endurance and strength together can limit muscle hypertrophy (growth) was popularized in a 1980 study. Over a 10-week period, researchers traced three groups of male respondents: the first group incorporated resistance training only, the second included cardio only (a combination of biking and running on the treadmill), and the third group incorporated both resistance training and cardio. The study concluded that training for strength and endurance simultaneously "reduced the capacity to develop strength."[3] However, this study is over four decades old, and the groups participating in cardio were doing it for six days a week (which is much more than what's typically recommended today).

More recent studies have shown that a moderate amount of cardio can *enhance* muscle growth in the gym. Quite the opposite of the 1980s study, but note the keyword *moderate*.

A 21-week study in 2012 observed the same three groups (strength only, endurance only, and strength and endurance) with *untrained* men, evaluating the impact each of these training programs had on their ability to grow muscle mass. The group that incorporated two days of endurance exercise and strength saw increases in muscle hypertrophy (growth); however, it's worth noting that the strength and endurance group's endurance efforts interfered with "explosive strength development, compared with strength and endurance training alone."[4] Simply put, some power or explosive movements in the gym might be hindered with cardio, but our body's ability to gain muscle isn't impacted by including some cardio in our weekly rotation.

IMPORTANT CARDIO FACTORS TO CONSIDER

Once again, we can't make a blanket statement about strength and endurance without diving deeper into the details. The type of cardio we do, the frequency, our training splits, the intensity, the duration of the activity, and factors like our genetics and others will all play a role in how cardio will affect our ability to build muscle. I think, for the sake of simplicity, it's better to separate out our training goals into two categories: bodybuilders (or those looking to maximize muscle gain and put on serious size) and everyone else (those who want to build some muscle but don't care to look like Dwayne "The Rock" Johnson).

This book isn't necessarily written for the first group but more so for the second. If you are looking to maximize muscle size in your lower body, the general consensus is to try to limit the amount of running or cycling you're doing, as it could impede muscle growth. But, and this is a big *but*, research shows that incorporating cardio doesn't seem to have much of an effect on our body's ability to gain or maintain upper-body muscle mass and strength at all.[5]

In addition, some scientific literature has emerged proving that running alone can build muscle, depending on both the intensity and duration. Sprinting versus long runs, for example, can have differing effects on our bodies.

One study put college students on a 10-week high-intensity interval training program. At the end of the program, the students saw increased muscle mass in their quads.[6] Sprinting can even enhance muscle protein synthesis: a key ingredient for our bodies to build muscle. On the other hand, long-distance running (> 10 kilometers/6.25 miles) can have the opposite effect. Long-distance running can cause damage to our muscles (especially as the mileage increases), which in turn could impede muscle growth.[7]

If you're doing copious amounts of cardio, it's important to keep an eye on your caloric intake and ensure that with the addition of extra exercise (which can be tracked in apps like MyFitnessPal), you're not exceeding a 20% deficit—otherwise, you risk losing muscle. If you're doing cardio and are still in a surplus or maintenance while on a progressive training plan, you shouldn't run into too many issues in your ability to gain lean muscle simultaneously. Now that we've debunked a few myths, let's move on to discuss types of cardio and the pros and cons of each.

LOW-INTENSITY STEADY-STATE VERSUS HIGH-INTENSITY INTERVAL TRAINING

Low-intensity steady-state (LISS) cardio is where we exercise at about 40–70% of our maximum heart rate. For example, walking or jogging at a light pace is LISS cardio. High-intensity interval training (HIIT) is short bursts of intense exercise interspersed with periods of low intensity and rest. Sprinting on the treadmill for intervals followed by a few minutes of walking or jogging or tempo run (running at or slightly below our lactate threshold) are examples of HIIT workouts.

Old schools of thought promoted LISS cardio, as it burns more fat during exercise than HIIT does. We now know the "crossover" effect where with low-intensity exercise, fat is the go-to source for fuel, whereas for higher intensity our bodies prioritize carbohydrates (glucose) for fuel. While this hypothesis makes sense on the surface, it's important to look at the effects not only *during* the session but *after* as well.

Newer schools of thought now say the opposite, that although low intensity does burn more fat during the exercise session than HIIT does, HIIT burns more calories *after* the session is over and continues to burn calories throughout the remainder of the day.

So which is more effective for fat loss? One of the determinants when comparing HIIT and LISS is post-exercise oxygen consumption—or how many calories we burn over a 24-hour period after exercising. Research has shown that HIIT requires a higher degree of oxygen consumption post-workout and therefore can burn more calories overall than LISS can. However, the number of calories burned at the end of the day wasn't significant enough to warrant choosing one type of cardio over the other.[8]

A 2017 meta-analysis took this even further and concluded that there were no differences between the two types on body fat reduction—both HIIT and moderate intensity aerobic exercise produced similar effects on body composition.[9]

Therefore, if choosing HIIT or LISS strictly for fat-loss purposes, either is a good option and warrants similar results. Let's look at some other pros and cons of each.

HIIT

Pros

- More time efficient—HIIT burns the same number of calories as LISS in less time
- Tends to be less boring than steady state
- Performance-wise, HIIT can improve our endurance and make us faster
- HIIT may reduce our appetite
- HIIT can potentially burn a few more calories throughout the day post-workout

Cons

- More difficult to recover from[10]
- Can be taxing and cut into our energy that we could be using toward our resistance training plan
- Pushing too hard can put us at a higher risk of an overuse injury

LISS

Pros

- LIIS feels much easier and is a more sustainable form of cardio over the long term
- Faster recovery post-workout

- LISS can be used as a form of active recovery on our rest days (improving blood flow, clearing lactic acid, and so on)
- Running or biking at a conversational pace can be an enjoyable activity to do with someone else
- Good for beginners who are just adopting an exercise regimen

Cons

- Not as time efficient as HIIT
- Can feel boring
- Once your body adapts to your LISS sessions, your body won't burn as many calories
- Your body stops burning calories once the session ends

Incorporating HIIT and LISS in Your Training

I recommend incorporating both HIIT and LISS into your workout depending on what your training plan is that day. I only include one to two HIIT workouts per week max (in the form of intervals on the treadmill or tempo/threshold runs). The rest of my aerobic exercise is in the form of steady-state cardio. How much you want to include depends on how fast you can recover from HIIT workouts, personal preferences, and what your training goals are. If you're looking to maximize muscle growth and strength, you may want to focus mostly on LISS, but one HIIT workout a week is a good idea too.

STRENGTH BEFORE CARDIO OR CARDIO BEFORE STRENGTH?

There isn't a ton of concrete evidence on which order is best, but most experts recommend prioritizing cardio or strength depending on your goals. If your goal is fat loss or gaining muscle (where most of us fall into), you'll want to start with resistance training first, followed by cardio. There is no direct correlation between muscle growth and the order of cardio and resistance training; the main variable here is energy. If you do a session of cardio at the beginning of your workout, you may feel wiped and your strength training therefore suffers.

If, however, you're like me and want to improve *aerobic* performance, you might want to prioritize cardio first. If I'm training for an upcoming race, I'll work on improving my running times. If I do strength beforehand, I won't be able to push myself as hard during those tough tempo or all-out runs. Here are some general guidelines based on my own unique goals to help me improve running times and build muscle (a.k.a. hybrid training):

- Upper-body days—resistance training before cardio

- Leg days—resistance training before cardio

- Core days—a HIIT workout first, and then core (my strength training sessions are shorter, so I don't need as much energy)

So you can mix and match depending on what you want to prioritize, but as a general rule, resistance training should come first and then cardio.

OPTIMAL AMOUNT OF CARDIO

Now that you know the types of cardio and the best order, what is the optimal amount of cardio you should include in your plan? You're going to love this answer: it depends! I would suggest incorporating two to four days of cardio per week broken out as follows:

- One to two HIIT sessions per week (20–30 minutes is usually sufficient): intervals on the treadmill or sprints on the bike

- Two to three LISS sessions per week (40 minutes to one hour per session): jogging at a light pace, easy work on the stationary bike, a casual bike ride, or walking

Thirty-minute sessions two to three times a week seem to be the sweet spot if you don't want to impede any of your lower-body muscle growth. However, if you don't care about building gigantic quads, include as much cardio as your little heart desires! If you think cardio is the devil, try for a minimum of two sessions and only do the LISS type. You don't have to do HIIT if you hate it; experiment with different types of cardio until you find a type you like. Remember, it's not so much the cardio that's important for fat loss; it's the nutrition aspect and keeping an eye on energy balance. Building muscle through resistance training is really going to move the mark in your body composition. The amount and type, therefore, can be at your discretion.

MY FAVORITE TREADMILL WORKOUT

Remember at the beginning of the book when I talked about that treadmill workout I found that changed my life? I've decided to include it in the book here because it made such a profound impact on me. This was the treadmill interval workout I used when I first started running—that helped me improve both pace and stamina over time (reflected on a US treadmill in miles per hour).

Minute 1: level 5 (12 min/mile pace)

Minute 2: level 6 (10 min/mile pace)

Minute 3: level 5

Minute 4: level 6

Minute 5: level 7 (8:34 min/mile pace)

Minute 6: level 5

Minute 7: level 6

Minute 8: level 7

Minute 9: level 8 (7:30 min/mile pace)

Minute 10: level 5

Minute 11: level 6

Minute 12: level 7

Minute 13: level 8

Minute 14: level 9 (6:40 min/mile pace)

Minute 15: level 5

Minute 16: level 6

Minute 17: level 7

Minute 18: level 8

Minute 19: level 9

Minute 20: level 10 (6 min/mile pace)

Minute 21: level 5 (cooldown)

Minute 22: level 5 (cooldown)

I think this is an amazing workout for beginners. You can adjust the levels as you see fit. Build up your endurance for short spurts, then rest and build it up again. You can start at level 3 (20 min/mile or walking pace) or 4 (15 min/mile or brisk walking pace). Over time, you'll be able to start at a much higher level. This is an example of what the first 22 minutes look like for me now:

Minute 1: level 7

Minute 2: level 8

Minute 3: level 8.5 (about 7:05 min/mile pace)

Minute 4: level 8.5

Minute 5: level 9

Minute 6: level 9

Minute 7: level 9

Minute 8: level 9

Minute 9: level 9.5

Minute 10: level 9.5

Minute 11: level 9

Minute 12: level 9

Minute 13: level 9.5

Minute 14: level 9.5

Minute 15: level 9.5

Minute 16: level 10

Minute 17: level 9

Minute 18: level 9

Minute 19: level 10

Minute 20: level 11 (5:27 min/mile pace)

Minute 21: level 8.5 (cooldown)

Minute 22: level 8.5 (cooldown)

The only difference between the two workouts is the speed and the fact that it's now 2021 and I've been doing intervals and treadmill workouts for 13 years.

PRACTICAL TRAINING TIPS TO MAXIMIZE RESULTS

Now that we've nailed down the training fundamentals, established some splits to choose from, and looked at what types of exercises we should focus on, let's go over some key training tips to help you maximize your results in the gym:

- Start with compound exercises before isolation.

- Train weaker points earlier in your workout (or in the week).

- Take the time to learn proper form—invest in a trainer or watch YouTube videos and practice the movements with lighter weights before lifting heavier.

- If you're not seeing the progress you want, you may not be putting forth enough effort in the gym. Make sure that on the last set of each exercise you're pushing so hard that you physically can't lift anymore (hitting technical failure). Try to train over 3 RIR or a 7 RPE most of the time.

- If you hit a plateau, try increasing the volume (add more sets or more weight).

- You want to make sure that when you're choosing each weight that it's not too light and not too heavy (a bit of trial and error is required here). Remember that you want to aim for the range we outlined based on the training application section.

- Tracking the reps and sets you're doing by pen and paper or an app will help you see your progression.

- For most of us, 6–15 reps is the ideal range we should aim for: below six and we may risk injury, and over 15 we may experience some issues with recovery and fatigue.

- A general rule of thumb is to prioritize resistance training before cardio.

- Incorporate both HIIT and LISS in your routine to improve performance and expedite fat loss.

CHAPTER 16

Tracking Your Progress

If you're new to training, the first few months of implementing a new plan is the time where you'll see body composition changes the quickest. As you get further along in your journey, you'll eventually hit a bit of a genetic ceiling (as I did). Changes in your body will be more incremental and you won't see significant changes in strength or muscle size. This is where details are important. When it comes to tracking your fitness progress, you should pay attention to the following four major items:

1. Calories

2. Protein

3. Body composition

4. Workouts (reps/sets/weekly volume)

We already covered ways to track calories and protein in Part II of the book. So in this section, we'll cover the best ways to track your body composition and your workouts.

BODY COMPOSITION

When you first think of tracking your progress in the gym, what comes to mind first? The scale, right? As we already covered, the scale can be deceiving and doesn't tell the whole story since our weight fluctuates quite a bit. So if you're going to track changes in weight, it's a good idea to track it daily, then take *weekly averages*. This will give you a general idea of whether week-over-week changes in your weight are going in the right or wrong direction. So, while you can certainly use the scale, don't use it as the main key performance indicator for your fitness goals.

Body fat percentage is much more indicative of progress than the scale, so if you have access at the gym to measure it, take advantage of it. If you don't have access to a fancy machine, you can visit a few different websites to get a guesstimate (https://rippedbody.com/body-fat-guide) or you can buy a body fat caliper.

Body fat scales, which are usually built into regular scales, aren't very accurate, so I don't recommend using them. Mine, for example, shows my body fat as 23%, and the machine at the gym shows 12%, which is quite the discrepancy.

Photo Journaling

Photo journaling, while highly analog and visual, is by far my favorite method to observe aesthetic improvements in my physique. It's especially good for beginners as a way to establish a baseline for comparing your progress against. Here's how it works: You'll want to strip down to your undies and take a photograph from the front, side, and back. Then you'll store the photos either in an app (MyFitnessPal, for example, keeps a photo diary with your respective weight) or you can use a spreadsheet or Word doc. I like keeping the photos in a spreadsheet and jotting down some notes below them. You can keep the photos side by side so you can compare and physically see what areas you're making the most progress in.

Measuring Tape

You can also choose to take body measurements with a regular measuring tape to track shrinkage/growth in key areas on your body. Or you can take measurements in conjunction with your photo journaling for extra details, and it's an easy (and inexpensive) way to go. You'll want to take measurements of your waist, chest, shoulders, hips, biceps, and thighs.

More Advanced Techniques

As you get more advanced in your training[1] and changes become more incremental, it's a good idea to become more meticulous with your training details by keeping a journal. Or you can use more advanced measures to get a fuller picture of your body composition. These devices are highly accurate and can provide more data than just your body fat percentage, such as body water, dry lean mass, body fat mass, lean body mass, skeletal mass, bone density, and so on. The drawback is that they can be pricey. Here are some popular devices to check out:

- *4C:* This is the most accurate and best method, as it measures body water. It's just not accessible to most and is also time consuming.

- *DEXA/XXA scan:* A popular and very accurate method. With DEXA, you're able to measure fat-free mass, fat mass, and bone density. It's a bit pricey, though, at around $125 a scan.

- *BodPod:* Provides data on fat-free mass and fat mass and is less expensive than DEXA. Still not the cheapest, but a BodPod test is around $45.

Aside from weight, you don't need to track all these other data on a day-to-day basis. Whichever method you use to track your body composition, weekly or even biweekly is just fine.

TRACKING WORKOUTS

I have a confession: I've never in the entirety of my fitness journey logged a single workout. Oops. Do I think it's a good idea? Yes, but I personally don't want to be plugging in my reps, sets, and exercises into a journal or app while working out. I prefer to stay present and focused on my workouts. I do have a rough idea of the weight and the reps I do for each of the exercises (a bit of a photographic memory), but I don't always remember the exact ranges. I simply focus on hitting muscle failure during each session on that very last set.

But I would be remiss to not suggest using some form of mechanism to track your workouts and progress in the gym. Keeping track of your reps/sets/volume per exercise can give you tangible metrics on whether you're getting stronger. If you do want to go this route, here are some of the best ways to track your progress:

- Create a training journal (reps/sets) per exercise each week.
- Use an app (e.g., Simple Workout Log, Gymaholic, or FitNotes).
- Input in a spreadsheet (e.g., Google Sheets, Pages, or Excel).

Let me be clear: tracking can be a good idea, but once again, it comes down to individualized preference. If tracking becomes too arduous and annoying, then it may become a deterrent, preventing us from showing up to our workouts. In my opinion, it's much better to show up more often and *enjoy our training* than meticulously track every aspect of our workout. Buyer beware.

DIFFERENCES IN OUR BODIES

As you track your progress, keep this thought in mind: Comparing ourselves and our progress to others can throw us into a negative tailspin. It's important to focus on your own training, your own progress, and your own body composition. Everyone's fitness journey is different, so don't get discouraged if you feel like others around you are making quicker progress.

On a similar note, I want to quickly address the fact that we all store fat in different places on our bodies and genetically, each of us is more adept at gaining muscle in specific areas over others. Unfortunately for us, and despite how much targeted training we do, losing weight isn't à la carte. We can't choose exactly where on our body we want to lose fat.

Some may carry weight in their lower body, some in their arms, and for me—I carry fat in my chest and stomach area. I've struggled over the years to get that "washboard ab" look. Despite training my entire body and applying the principles outlined in this book, I was seeing minimal progress with the extra weight on my stomach. My legs and arms got leaner, my boobs shrunk a bit (wah), but my body fat took out a second mortgage on my stomach.

Spot treatment—picking and choosing where we lose body fat by doing highly targeted exercises—is a myth. While you can certainly increase the likelihood of your muscles showing in particular areas if you train and apply the principles of progressive overload, that doesn't mean they're going to "pop" like you see with fitness models. You're going to need to lower your body fat percentage significantly enough to see the muscles show through.

The fact is, if we want to get the "shredded" look, then we need to get our body fat down. This is particularly true with showing those elusive six-pack abdominal muscles. From physique coach Paul Revelia's experience, he notes, "For women to get on the leaner side, it requires getting around 15–17% body fat, whereas for men, they need to get down to around 10% to see their abs for the most part. If women get under the 10% mark, that look is extremely shredded."[2] Under 15%, as mentioned earlier, is not recommended or healthy for cis women to sustain.

Just realize that the differences in our gender and genetics will play a role in how fast we progress, where we build muscle the fastest, and which areas of our body we'll lose fat first.

TAKEAWAYS

I'm asking you to track a lot of things, and it can get a bit tedious and overwhelming. I personally don't like logging every detail of my workout and don't use a measuring tape. What I recommend is choosing methods for tracking your body composition and training that are manageable and that you'll actually keep up with. Only you know yourself and how much admin work you can stomach before getting annoyed and bogged down.

CHAPTER 17

The Importance of Sleep

We all know how important sleep is to our overall health, but what some people don't realize is the extent to which sleep can stymie our progress (if we don't get sufficient amounts of it). Even if you're following your training and nutrition to a tee, you might not see the results moving in the right direction if you're not getting enough shut-eye. Here's how lack of sleep can sabotage our training and nutrition plans.

INCREASED APPETITE AND POOR FOOD CHOICES

Studies have shown that lack of sleep results in a stronger appetite because of increases in the hormone ghrelin and decreases in leptin.[1] Point blank—an increased appetite leads to overeating (and poorer food choices), which leads to weight gain.

Ghrelin is known as the hunger hormone because it stimulates our appetite. It's produced in our gut, and its main role is to make us hungry so that we eat more. Ghrelin travels through our bloodstream all the way up to the brain and sends signals to the hypothalamus (a part of our brain the controls appetite) that it's hungry.[2] *"Feed me,"* says ghrelin. Ghrelin often increases when we're dieting or in a caloric deficit for prolonged periods, but inadequate sleep is also a main trigger for increases in this hormone.

Remember our other good friend leptin back in the nutrition part of the book? To refresh our memory, leptin is also known as the satiety hormone—it's released by our fat cells and tells the hypothalamus that we're full. High levels of leptin send signals that we're satiated, whereas low levels cause us to feel famished. Basically, leptin is a survival mechanism that tells our brain if we have sufficient fat to survive.

One study observed over 1,000 participants and the number of hours of sleep they got each night. Researchers found that those who slept less than eight hours saw proportionally lower levels of leptin and increased levels of ghrelin.[3]

When we have adequate sleep, we feel better, more alert, we have more self-control, and have the ability to make smarter choices with our food.[4] On the other hand, a lack of sleep can decrease our decision-making ability and increase our appetite. Less willpower is a likely side effect, and chances are, we'll opt for food options that (a) lack nutritional value and (b) are more calorie dense—to satisfy our seemingly insatiable hunger.[5]

I don't know about you, but I've experienced this so many times. Here's a play-by-play on what a typical sleep-deprived day looks like for me: I feel foggy headed, lazy, sluggish, unproductive, and no matter how much I eat, I can't seem to get full. Studies have also shown that the reward center in our brains is more heightened with food when we lack sleep, once again causing us to overeat and sabotaging our fat-loss efforts.[6]

NEGATIVE IMPACTS ON OUR TRAINING

Bad sleep can completely sabotage our training. This is an obvious one. If you're tired, you're not going to be able to put your all into your workouts and push through those hard sets (hitting RPE > 7 or RIR < 3) that are vital for muscle growth. We've all experienced that lagging energy and lack of motivation at the gym. It's okay if you have a few bad nights—you're not always going to get beautiful, restful sleep and jump out of bed like a spring chicken. But when it happens often or, worse, chronically, that's when you're really going to see the deleterious effects on your training efforts.

Similarly, your resting metabolic rate (RMR) is responsible for burning calories while you're at rest, and some studies have shown that lack of sleep can cause your RMR to decrease.[7] Other studies have also shown that lack of sleep can lead to muscle loss—something we definitely want to avoid.[8]

OTHER ISSUES

Chronic (longer-term) lack of sleep can lead to insulin resistance and even type 2 diabetes.[9] Not prioritizing sleep can also lead to other negative impacts on our mood, blood pressure, and immune system (making us more susceptible to illness and disease) and can cause anxiety, stress, and even depression. In our work, lack of sleep makes us feel less motivated and focused.

THE OPTIMAL AMOUNT OF SLEEP

By now, it should be clear that lack of sleep can be a big determinant in stunting our fitness progress—aesthetically and performance-wise. So how much sleep do we really need? Of course, there are outliers, but the overwhelming scientific literature suggests if you're between 18 and 64, you need seven to nine hours of sleep, and adults over 65 years may need a bit less (seven to eight hours).[10] Some need more sleep than others. Athletes, for example, might need even more than nine hours. It's normal after running a marathon to crash for several hours post-race. You know how you feel when you're tired, so try to prioritize at least seven to eight hours, and maybe even more.

TIPS TO GETTING A GOOD NIGHT'S SLEEP

I've had troubles with sleep since my childhood and still struggle with it today. Actually, I think it's gotten worse as I've aged. I need to sleep with a fan noise every night. The white noise is so loud, you could easily mistake it for a car engine. Over the years, I've tried to tweak my bedtime routine to get more restful sleeps. It's not foolproof, but the following tips may help you get a bit better quality shut-eye:

- Turn your phone on airplane mode at night, or if you have the will-power, stop looking at your phone an hour before bedtime. Research has shown that the blue light your phone emits affects your circadian rhythm.[11]

- Limit caffeine intake throughout the day (the amount you consume depends on tolerance)—try not to consume any caffeine at least six hours before bedtime.[12] I would go as far as to say eight hours. I personally don't drink any coffee past 1:00 p.m. for my 10:00 p.m. bedtime, or else it affects my sleep. Some rare specimens, like my dad, can drink coffee a few hours before bed and sleep soundly. I don't know how. For the general population (myself included), try to avoid those afternoon caffeine hits.

- Read before bed. Reading helps us relax and makes us sleepy. I personally read for around an hour or so (sometimes more, sometimes less), until my brain stops absorbing the information and I can transition soundly into sleep.

- Avoid alcohol before bedtime—while some alcohol can knock us out and help us fall asleep fast, the actual quality of our sleep is terrible when we drink.[13]

- Be mindful of what you eat before bed—a high-carb meal right before bedtime might give us a glucose spike and energy. A big meal too close to bedtime not only is uncomfortable but can also disrupt sleep from ingestion. On the opposite side of the spectrum, going to bed hungry can also be uncomfortable. I personally like to eat a high-protein snack (about 150–200 calories) before bed either in the form of a whey protein shake or a protein bar. Some studies have shown that consuming a bit of protein before bed can help with overnight muscle protein synthesis.[14]

- Sleeping in the cold is better than hot for a restful sleep. Our body temperatures drop when we're sleeping, so the colder temps can help regulate our temperatures. Studies have shown that about 65°F or 18°C is the ideal temperature range for sleep.[15]

Training, nutrition, and sleep are the three key ingredients to our body recomp pie. If we're lagging in any of the three areas, we won't be able to reach our potential in the gym and our efforts may be moot. So, as with training and nutrition, *prioritize your sleep*, and make tweaks to ensure you're receiving adequate amounts. I end this section with a quotation from Matthew Walker in *Why We Sleep*:

> AMAZING BREAKTHROUGH! Scientists have discovered a revolutionary new treatment that makes you live longer. It enhances your memory and makes you more creative. It makes you look more attractive. It keeps you slim and lowers food cravings. It protects you from cancer and dementia. It wards off colds and the flu. It lowers your risk of heart attacks and stroke, not to mention diabetes. You'll even feel happier, less depressed, and less anxious. Are you interested?[16]

The treatment, by the way, is sleep.

PART IV

————————

SUSTAINABILITY

CHAPTER 18

Progress over the Long Term

We should now be equipped with the knowledge and tools to make radical changes to our bodies, mindset, and overall health—but knowledge may not be enough. Progress can be painfully slow at times and it's discouraging. We map out our training splits and nutrition plans meticulously until a big life event happens: we lose our job, we lose a family member or close friend, or we suffer from our own health issues. We fall off our plan. We stop making progress. We find it infinitely more difficult to start back up and get in a groove again.

Sustainability practices are the last part of the book, but equally important to your mindset, nutrition, and training. This is an ongoing, lifelong process. Only you can decide the role you want fitness to play in your life.

As I mention in the fitness goals chapter, if and when you hit your body recomposition goals, there comes a point in time where you'll be thinking, *What's next? Where do I go from here?*

Fitness has played such a key role in my life for so long—it keeps me grounded and makes me happy. I've been able to sustain a consistent routine for over 13 years now, and as I write this, I've run an average of 10 kilometers a day every day for over four years. I would never have been able to sustain my everyday practice if I only framed my training as a weight-loss tool—to achieve an egocentric goal or obtain an aesthetic look or to prove to others that I'm worthy. I've been able to discover much *deeper* reasons why I train based on how it makes me *feel*.

In Part IV, I cover some of the main keys to sustainability: defining success and your long-term progress, how to deal with the inevitable (and dreaded plateaus), dealing with the bad days, prioritizing your self-care, and using your support system to help you stick with your commitments. I conclude with a few warnings on what to look out for in your fitness journey and briefly touch on how a meditation practice can enhance and bring more joy to your training.

DEFINING SUCCESS

First, how do you define success with your fitness goals? What does that look like for you? While we now know that goals provide a good direction for our efforts, the daily actions should be our focal point—to define that success. I encourage you, once again, to move away from aesthetics as the sole driver of your efforts and to derive other benefits from fitness—that's inclusive of all types of movement. Personal trainer and motivational coach Lauren Leavell writes, "One of my favorite reasons to continue building endurance and strength is to be able to move furniture on my own. Without help. Whenever I want."[1] For me, having the ability to walk over half a mile home with two big bags of groceries as a result of my strength training is liberating.

Michelle Segar suggests using a low-end and high-end range of what she calls "the continuum of success." She writes, "Research shows that people are more successful at achieving their goals when they can choose from a range of low-end and high-end goals rather than aiming at one specific goal."[2]

A low-end goal could be doing lower volume in the gym, cleaning the house, mowing the lawn, hitting one body part, or walking instead of running. A high-end goal could be hitting your volume goals (sets and reps in a given workout) or incorporating the high-intensity interval training

(HIIT) session you had planned. Anything else that falls in the middle is considered a success. You can pat yourself on the back for showing up and doing something.

CONSISTENCY TRUMPS INTENSITY. PERIOD.

Sustainability and consistency go hand in hand. Intensity should be used sparingly, since it runs counter to consistency.

Many people throw in the towel too soon. They approach their workouts with high intensity for short durations, don't see the results right away, and feel like their efforts are wasted. Honestly, I don't blame them. If I approached my everyday workouts knowing they would be akin to a punishment—sweat pouring off of me, feeling like I'm on the verge of puking (or actually puking)—then I would rarely, if ever, step foot in a gym. If I continuously held the image of a woman (me) gasping for air, soaked in sweat, I wouldn't last long.

Gently remind yourself that you're in this for the long haul. Most of my workouts are easy. In fact, over 80% of my runs are at a conversation pace, at which I could talk on the phone simultaneously. I only incorporate HIIT or tempo runs (holding challenging or "comfortably hard" paces for prolonged periods of time) once or twice a week maximum. If I push myself too hard when my body or mind isn't feeling it, I'll be more susceptible to injury or risk experiencing burnout. My goal is to keep up my consistent running streak and be able to integrate training into my everyday life. There's no way I'd be able to achieve this if I went full throttle, Dwayne Johnson–style, seven days a week.

One way to achieve consistency in your fitness plan is through the act of compounding. This principle does not apply just to the interest accumulated over time on our investments; it applies to every aspect of our lives. Small actions every single day accumulate and materialize into massive changes over time. The habits that we develop today will eventually help shape the person we become over the long term.

It's hard to stick to an action every day when we don't feel like we're moving forward—when we feel like we're at a standstill. Until one day—maybe months, maybe years down the road—we see our efforts materialize into real progress that we never thought possible. James Clear calls this the "plateau of latent potential." He writes, "When you finally break through the Plateau of Latent Potential, people will call it an overnight success."[3] I remember the first time I saw a vein emerge in my bicep. I wondered how that happened. Then I remembered that I had been lifting weights for over two years. I also didn't emerge out of the womb as a runner; I picked it up later in life and slowly became better over time. I would never have been able to run 74 consecutive half marathons without a solid base. I had been running regularly for almost 10 years—finishing several half marathons and marathons (plus the consecutive 10K/31-day challenge) before embarking on this much larger challenge. Compounding is the opposite of instant gratification—the payoff of our efforts is delayed for long periods of time. But as we become more competent and pay attention to little victories, compounding provides a new burst of motivation and energy to keep going.

DITCH THE "ALL OR NOTHING" MENTALITY

I've fallen prey to many of the following "all or nothing" mentality statements too many times: "If I don't hit a certain amount of mileage, it doesn't count," or "If I'm not profusely sweating after exercise, it doesn't count," or "If I don't work out for a specific amount of time, it doesn't count," or "If I don't follow my nutrition plan to a tee, then it doesn't count."

This type of thinking runs counter to the principle of compounding. It prevents you from taking the essential incremental steps each day to improve yourself—not only with your training but with every skill you want to develop in life. This attitude kills progress—impeding the material gains that crystallize from the compounding of small efforts over time. Putting yourself in a rigid box can strip away motivation, cause procrastination, and reinforce the idea that no matter what we do, it's not enough. You might strive to fulfill the increasingly high standards you set for yourself. This is especially true for people with type A personalities, like me.

Switching our mentality to *everything counts* is a more sustainable approach to our goals; we can celebrate our victories despite how seemingly small they are. When I switched my thinking to "everything counts," I was satisfied doing less mileage in a day. I was content with doing low-intensity exercise at a slower pace. I felt a sense of accomplishment for simply showing up and doing something—especially on the days where I had zero energy and felt like garbage.

Remember that any movement or action, any piece of food we eat that energizes us, any form of exercise (even just a walk or a casual bike ride) counts toward making progress on your goals. We're not going to see our body change from a single or even a handful of workouts. Studies have shown repeatedly that positive reinforcement promotes sustainable behavior change. Adopt the mentality that any small change counts toward your goals, and you're well on your way to obtaining a sustainable fitness regimen for life.

CHAPTER 19

Overcoming the Plateau and Dealing with Bad Days

No matter where you are in your training, you will eventually hit the inevitable and dreaded plateau. A plateau is where the progress we're making slows down significantly or comes screeching to a halt. Our bodies acclimate to stressors, and changes become incremental or visibly nonexistent. Plateaus can be performance-related or body composition–related. For instance, we run our slowest time on our five-mile route (in months), the same weight we squatted last week feels more difficult, or we don't see as much muscle growth or any real aesthetic changes week over week. Sometimes, we may even regress and lose a bit of muscle mass.

Plateaus are discouraging but quite common; they happen to all of us. Beginners always make progress the fastest, which is exciting and motivating, but when the stall comes rolling around, it can be disheartening. As we progress and changes become increasingly incremental, we're even more likely to experience a plateau. In this section, I go over a few strategies on how to identity when you've hit a plateau and what to do about it.

First things first. If you hit a plateau, don't panic. Self-compassion is important here because if you start chastising yourself, it's only going to be a deterrent to your journey. If your goal is fat loss, realize that our bodies' process of adaptive thermogenesis is probably playing a role. As you continue to lose weight and decrease your body fat percentage, your body will want to hold on to those fat stores for dear life—it's a survival mechanism. This process is likely to occur if you're in a caloric deficit for too long and experience decreases in your metabolism. Also realize that eventually you'll hit a bit of a ceiling when it comes to naturally building muscle (as mentioned earlier).

REVIEW YOUR FITNESS PLAN

First off, plan that a plateau is going to happen. This sounds obvious, but if you somehow think you're some godlike specimen who will never experience basic laws of human nature, well, you're in for a rude awakening. This is where details become important. Take a step back and try to get a holistic view on all the moving parts of your training, nutrition, and recovery plan. Ask yourself the following questions:

- What's my current calorie intake? Has my body adapted to the new weight? Is it time to recalculate?

- Am I hitting my protein targets?

- Am I getting enough sleep?

- Am I possibly overtraining and not incorporating enough rest days? Look for signs of overtraining syndrome (OTS): mental and physical exhaustion, prolonged periods of soreness and pain, and ongoing bad moods.

- Am I applying the principles of progressive overload and exerting enough effort and intensity in my workouts to hit muscle failure? Am I training at a RPE greater than 7 or RIR less than 3 most of the time?

After you've reviewed your plan, you might want to go back to tracking more meticulous details if you've stopped (counting calories, protein intake, and begin logging your workouts—reps/sets/weekly volume per muscle group) to see if you can find any low-hanging fruit to adjust in your plan. Then make one or two small changes and see what happens over the course of a week or two. Don't go changing a million variables at once, as tempting as that is. Here are some ideas on what you can change in your workout to help you move forward and break through a plateau:

- Adjust your calorie intake—if you've been in a deficit for too long, incorporate a refeed day or two or contemplate a diet break.

- Try mixing up your routine—incorporate a new exercise, mix up the order of your exercises, or test out a different training split.

- Add another rest day to your routine.

"Progress is non-linear," writes Brad Stulberg, cocreator of the *Growth Equation*.[1] You may feel like you are taking one step forward, two steps back, and one step sideways before you see progress. Sometimes it's not so much a matter of making all these changes to your routine but, rather, continuing to show up and push through the plateau. Eventually, you'll come out of it.

TACKLING BAD DAYS

Just like we need to accept and plan for the plateau, we also need to acknowledge that bad days are going to happen—you may feel lethargic, have low energy, or simply have a crap workout. Procrastination, or what Steven Pressfield calls "the Resistance,"[2] is at an all-time high. We're finding it harder and harder to get off the couch or out of bed and out the door. Simply put, we just don't *feel* like it. Let me tell you a secret: I often don't *feel* like it either. Even after sustaining a routine for over 13 years, I still experience bad days. Sometimes they only last part of the day, sometimes the whole day, and sometimes for weeks at a time. In short, it sucks. Ladies, this is especially true around our period, right? I'm sure you know what I'm talking about. The last thing I want to do is work out when I feel like a T-Rex is clawing at my uterus and my boobs feel like sandbags.

Even if you are in the worst mood, one of the best methods to improve your mood is to *take action*. Focus on how your training makes you feel during and after your workout. Those first few minutes of my workout are always the hardest. Nine times out of 10, when I get going, I start to feel better and get into that flow state in which I'm working out and time just disappears. I'm not focused on the time that elapsed on the treadmill or looking down at my Garmin at how many miles I've clocked. I'm simply being present with the workout: focusing on my breath and feeling that lovely burning sensation in my muscles after doing some hard sets.

It's getting our bums in gear and meandering out the door that's the hard part. Psychologists prescribe a therapy that involves taking action for people diagnosed with clinical depression called behavioral activation—part of cognitive behavioral therapy (CBT). Basically, the lower you're feeling—and experiencing negative emotions such as depression, apathy, anger, anxiety, loneliness—and the less motivated you are to do something, the more important it is to take action and physically move your body. Many of us are inclined to wait until we have motivation or energy to do something, but the emotions surrounding anxiety and depression are what one research paper states will make us want to "avoid and isolate."[3] The lower you're feeling (depressed, apathetic, angry, anxious), the harder it's going to be to pull yourself out of that state on your own or in a place of rest.

However, if you *physically move*, once you start the activity (a run or even get to the gym and do your first set), you'll notice something almost immediately—your mood begins to change. Exercise causes actual chemical changes in our brains. John J. Ratey writes:

> Going for a run is like taking a little bit of Prozac and a little bit of Ritalin because, like the drugs, exercise elevates these neurotransmitters. [Exercise] *balances* neurotransmitters—along with the rest of the neurochemicals in the brain.[4]

These chemicals make us *feel good*. The more we repeat this behavior over time and develop positive experiences from moving, the more discipline we develop and the easier it becomes over time to follow the same patterns. The technical term is called "reinforcing positive context contingencies." The University of Michigan authors of one paper, "Behavioral Activation for Depression," explain, "Research has shown that our decision to activate (in other words, to do the opposite of what the depression wants us to do, and do something in line with our values and goals) is necessary for emotions to change."[5]

When you have an inclination to take action, move right away. Mel Robbins, in her popular book *The 5 Second Rule*, suggests that as soon as you have an impulse to do something—to act on a particular goal—take action right away, within five seconds, to be exact. Otherwise, your brain will likely talk you out of it.[6] Controlling our emotions through action is one of the most effective strategies for dealing with the bad days.

FALLING OFF THE PATH

Aside from the plateaus and bad days, sometimes you may fall completely off the path. When this occurs, the frequency of missed workouts increases, and you may revert back to your old eating behaviors or stop working out altogether. A major crisis or life event happened (a death in the family, the birth of a child, for example), you are burned out from all the added stressors of life (we took on too much at once), or perhaps we're simply fatigued from our training and nutrition regimen—it's gotten boring. Once we start seeing ourselves slip and revert back to old behaviors, there's a tendency to chastise ourselves and thus reinforce the negative behaviors. Rather than foster negative emotions, which will only fuel the fire and downward spiral, it's important to take a step back—outside yourself—and develop and practice self-compassion.

WHAT IS SELF-COMPASSION?

Dr. Kristen Neff defines self-compassion as a reaction to one's suffering or "personal mistakes, perceived inadequacies, or various experiences of life difficulty."[7] Neff breaks self-compassion into three components:

1. *Mindfulness:* Having the conscious awareness of our thoughts and emotions. We can observe negativity toward ourselves and let go of the self-deprecation instead of ruminating or identifying with negative thoughts and emotions.

2. *Self-kindness:* When we experience negative thoughts on our own self-worth, we meet these emotions with care and kindness over criticizing and chastising ourselves.

3. *Common humanity:* Realizing that suffering and our human imperfection are universal—not uniquely tied to our own circumstance.[8]

SELF-COMPASSION AND ADHERENCE TO EXERCISE

A mindfulness practice is one of the keys to helping cope with the incessant negative chatter and self-deprecating thoughts your mind might feed you on an ongoing basis. If you miss a workout, don't listen to what your mind might be telling you: I'm a failure, I can't stick to anything, I'm worthless, and so on. Observe this mind chatter and choose to disengage.

As an alternative, replace the negative talk with curiosity and ask: Why am I missing my workouts? Why am I reverting back to old behaviors? Do some journaling and inner work to get to the real root of the issue. Perhaps you have too much on your plate right now and need to rebalance priorities, or you're not enjoying your workouts like you used to. Maybe you are focused too much on extrinsic rewards or external validation.

A study from the University of Manitoba and University of Ottawa looked at the role self-compassion plays on self-regulation (or in other words, self-discipline) on exercise following a setback. In line with the self-determination theory (that Part I discusses), the participants who originally set exercise goals from an intrinsic perspective (self-mastery, to feel good, etc.) were more likely to express self-compassion than those of their extrinsic goal counterparts—those who exercised because they should or out of obligation, ego-driven, or "social physique anxiety."[9] The study also found that the intrinsic group ruminated less on negative emotions and had higher levels of goal reengagement. In other words, they were able to get back on the path faster than those focusing on outward goals. Intrinsic motivation combined with practicing self-compassion can help reengage faster after you experience a setback.[10]

PRACTICING SELF-COMPASSION

Ruminating on negative experiences is exhausting. If you're stuck too long in this period, it can completely drain the energy you could be using to instead get yourself back in the game. Imperfection is a shared human experience; on this journey you'll experience setbacks and plateaus and *fall off* at some point. You may have stretches where you won't see any palpable results because life will happen and throws you off course. We're human beings, not bionic machines. When you build the foundation, however, you will develop the strength and self-discipline to get back on course and keep going. If you lose a battle, remember that life is a war. There will always be more internal battles to win. Self-compassion is a big work in progress for me too. Just be kind to yourself; it's that simple.

CHAPTER 20

Prioritizing Yourself

Another big road block to sustainability in fitness is this whole idea behind prioritization. When life happens—we have a baby, enter into a new relationship, start a new business, or begin a demanding job—our self-care can sometimes take the back seat. We need to take a step back and shift our priorities. More often than not, exercise is pushed down lower on that list and, if we're not careful, can be omitted altogether.

Fitness and health are two of the most important components of your life; if we're not physically healthy, nothing else matters. We won't be able to perform at our jobs, care for our family, give our best to our relationships. That's why reminding ourselves of the vital roles training, nutrition, and sleep have on our well-being is so important. Like sleep, exercise is akin to a magic pill—it can help with depression, anxiety, and sadness. It can prevent and even cure some diseases. However, it's not a one-and-done type deal; the pill needs to be taken regularly—for our whole life—to build and sustain the positive side effects.

When you're physically fit and healthy—whatever that looks like for you—you exude confidence. You have more energy to be present with your family and in your relationships. You have more focus and can more easily get into the elusive flow state at work or in your creative pursuits. Reminding yourself often of the benefits of exercise and not compromising on this time you set aside for yourself is key to sustainability.

Contingency planning can help us deal with life circumstances that come expectedly or unexpectedly our way. For instance, if you are about to have a child, your life is going to change, no doubt. You'll have to work with your partner on rearranging your schedule—compromising on when you can fit time in for you. If you're a single parent, perhaps working out from home is a better option. I've seen new parents bring their babies to the gym in their stroller—I love that so much. If you're used to working out right after work but now have a work schedule where you need to work later hours, try finding a way to squeeze in that workout before or during your lunch break. Even if it's just going for a walk or light jog, remember folks, everything counts. When I was traditionally employed, I used to run to work—saving time and money commuting, while getting in a workout. The key here is to be creative and plan. If you really want to prioritize your workouts, you'll make it work.

BENEFITS OF EXERCISE

If someone tries to talk you out of taking care of yourself, show them the following list. You should never have to justify or rationalize taking care of your health to anyone. Certain people or demanding jobs will try to vie for your time. It's important, therefore, to protect this time; set boundaries and share why you are not willing to compromise on taking this time for yourself every day (if you want to). I don't live in a fantasy world where I think we all have an abundance of time and can freely structure our days however we wish; you probably don't either. The world has real demands on our time and energy. Understanding the role exercise plays in our lives and how it can make us a holistically healthier, more productive, and happier individual will help us to better protect this time.

Several studies have shown the effects aerobic exercise has on positive cognitive outcomes. Working out can improve academic performance, can increase the rate of learning, can improve complex problem-solving skills, and has been proven in several school settings to increase focus on cognitive tasks in children. Adults can reap the same rewards, and studies have also shown that aerobic exercise can slow down the aging of our brain; both short term and long term, aerobic exercise contributes to overall brain health.[1] The following are some of the many other science-backed benefits of exercise. It:

- Helps reduce symptoms of depression in some cases

- Helps reduce anxiety

- Promotes a more positive outlook on life

- Reduces stress

- Changes chemicals in your brain to improve learning skills

- Helps you stay more focused and attentive at work

- Helps you sleep better at night

- Fosters a sense of community and belonging—through classes, team sports, and running groups, for instance

- Prevents some disease and illness

- Strengthens your immune system

PRODUCTIVE TRAINING

If this list doesn't suffice and you still feel some guilt for taking time out of your day to perform a self-care activity—something I still struggle with—try using your training sessions productively or what I call *productive training*. When I have a busy day at work but want to fit in a 1.5- to 2-hour workout with some strength training and a longer run, for instance, I plan activities that I can do while I work out to minimize the guilt of taking care of myself. I listen to a nonfiction audiobook when I run (so I'm learning), I take a meeting while walking on the treadmill or outdoors, or I answer emails while I'm on the stationary bike. Most importantly, the attentional space I'm giving myself during my workouts *is work*. I am actively working on piecing together sentences for my book, coming up with a solution to a difficult client problem, or simply coming up with new topic ideas to write about. Aside from my early morning hours when my brain is the most alert, working out is my second-most productive time of the day. "It's time we started considering physical activity as part of the work itself," writes psychologist Ron Friedman in *Harvard Business Review*.[2] While there isn't much research yet, some studies have shown that exercise can help bolster creativity.

We've all caught wind of inspirational anecdotes about how the "greats" used exercise to help with creative flow. To fuel his writing, Charles Dickens walked for three hours a day, carrying his notepad with him. Steve Jobs held walking meetings around Apple's headquarters in Cupertino, California. Best-selling author Ryan Holiday runs because he believes it makes him stronger at his job, explaining that "running is predictable, dependable, satisfying and thus a counterbalance for the mercurial muses of the creative professional."[3]

I've been using this strategy more recently with my creative work. I use my training as a way to problem solve and brainstorm on the creative projects I'm working on. This strategy is similar to object meditation where you pose a question and focus on the answers during your practice.

Using your training for other pursuits—not just self-care—can help you make your workouts a higher priority in life. This just adds even more fuel to the intrinsic fire—keeping the fire burning strong and helping us keep fitness in our lives over the long run.

FAMILY AND RELATIONSHIPS

While my relationship, job, and family situation isn't the same as yours, I've been in relationships before in which my partner wasn't supportive of my training regimen. My training is a time I protect wholeheartedly, and I've left relationships obviously not just for this reason but because my partner held me back in other areas of self-growth in my life as well. In this failed relationship, I realized that this person was not a full match for me. Yes, when you enter a relationship, some flexibility is involved, but there should be things in your life you're willing to compromise on and some that you aren't.

If you're in a relationship or have a family, talk to your partner and let them know that you want to start or uphold a training program. If there's resistance, explain the benefits and how you'll be able to show up and be a better partner and/or parent. Your partner and family should be supportive, but you can also get them involved too. Who knows, maybe your spouse/partner might start accompanying you on your runs or to the gym. You can make exercising a healthy and fun new activity together (check out the next section on accountability partners).

FIND AN ACCOUNTABILITY PARTNER

Once the initial euphoria and excitement wears off after starting a new regimen, you're now left with just the plain old hard work. And I'm not going to lie; training can be boring, arduous, and monotonous at times. Establishing habits and intrinsic motivation toward our training programs are two prerequisites for sustainability, but if we incorporate people in our fitness journey, our chances of sticking with our commitments go up exponentially.

Over the past few years, I've scheduled weekly calls with my good friend when not only do we catch up on life and work, but our main agenda item is to check in with each other on our goals. Kristie is one of the most disciplined and hardest-working people I know. If she sets a goal for herself, she's laser focused on achieving it and will persevere until it's accomplished. For instance, on a Thursday, she told me she was leaving her job as the vice president of marketing at a tech company. By that Saturday, she had already signed up for and begun a course on how to start a coaching company. The same afternoon, she had crafted almost a full first draft of her business plan and also calculated her financial plan to give her a runway for six months to get her new business started. I love this about Kristie, and it is why I chose her as my accountability partner.

An accountability partner is someone you can check in with regularly to do what the name implies: keep you accountable to the commitments you set for yourself. Scheduling regular calls or in-person check-in meetings can help you make faster progress. If you find someone who is pursuing similar goals, they can help you generate ideas to get you back on track (if you fall off) or share similar experiences and what they did to overcome them. You need an accountability partner not just for your fitness and nutrition but for other goals in life as well. In fact, Kristie is writing her own book, and checking in with her regularly helped me navigate the crazy world of book writing and figure out my own writing process.

Be careful when you're choosing someone. You'll want to find a partner who supports you and wants to see you grow and isn't afraid to be candid with you because they have your best interest at heart. Someone who is also driven, ambitious, and has personal goals of their own. If you find someone who's achieved something you want to achieve, even better because they can act as a mentor and help you to achieve your goals.

Sharing your goals with others can expose vulnerability and open the doors to judgment and critique. Working with a supportive accountability partner will help move you to action by providing gentle encouragement, which can foster more self-confidence and quiet the self-deprecating voices.

MAKE IT SOCIAL

Remember back to SDT theory that relatedness, or the way we feel connected and can relate to others, is a form of intrinsic motivation that can help us achieve our goals. Research has shown that fostering a sense of community and belonging can better help us stick to a fitness regimen. Going for a run or to the gym with a friend, joining a sports team, or signing up for a fitness class can all help foster a sense of community. We get to expand the individual benefits and make our training social. While my workouts are mostly individual (I enjoy my alone time), I do occasionally like to go for runs with others and love playing team sports.

CHAPTER 21

Adopting a Meditation and Mindfulness Practice

Most books in the health and fitness realm will recommend adopting a meditation practice. However, when I first read this advice, on a surface level, I wasn't able to make the habit stick. I didn't understand why I was sitting alone in silence, focusing on my breath. My practice was inconsistent, and when I did force myself to do it, I could only handle a few minutes at a time because of my lack of understanding of the actual context surrounding the practice.

When researching this book, I saw that most fitness/health authors recommended a meditation practice, but what I didn't see often was an explanation of the real reasons *why you should practice.* Learning to sit in a lotus position and focus on breathing and watching your thoughts is one thing, but this didn't help me adopt a practice because it didn't provide any meaning to me. If there isn't more context involved and the applicability of the practice on your personal goals, it isn't easy to prioritize other activities and sustain them over the long term. *Shouldn't I be doing something else more productive?* The mind will say, *I'm not progressing, so what's the point?*

I didn't know if I was correctly doing the practice. In fact, I thought I was doing it wrong and chastised myself a lot of the time during my meditation. I created negative experiences and associations with the practice. I felt like an amateur and didn't see myself improving in any capacity. It was discouraging.

After failing to stick with my practice consistently, I sought out new resources to help me. I read every meditation book I could get my hands on: Eckhart Tolle's *The Power of Now*, Tara Brach's *Radical Acceptance*, Michael Singer's *The Untethered Soul* and *The Surrender Experiment*, Sogyal Rinpoche's *The Tibetan Book of the Living and Dying*, and David Hawkins's *Letting Go*, among many others. I also started doing guided meditations with apps like Headspace and Calm and discovered Tara Brach's incredible meditation podcast on Spotify. I finally started learning the ropes and understanding the applicability, which, in turn, gave my practice much more meaning and practicality to my daily life.

Then I really upped my game. I became a student under a *shifu* (master) and started putting in the ongoing inner work to make transformational changes in my life. Attending classes at a Buddhist temple in Toronto, in a group setting, provided a whole new type of experience. My shifu trained in China at the famous Shaolin Temple and became a master in kung fu, tai chi, and meditation. His teachings helped me make transformative changes in my inner life and altered how I experienced setbacks, shortcomings, and challenges.

In this chapter, I do not teach you how to do meditation; there are many more resources and spiritual practitioners who are much more qualified than I am on this subject. However, what I share is the context for a meditation practice and how it can help you stick to your training and nutrition plan over the long term. And, more importantly, how learning to be mindful and fully present while you eat and train can bring you much more enjoyment in your life.

MEDITATION IN A NUTSHELL

In a very rudimentary Cliffs/Coles Notes version, meditation is simply returning to your roots; it's reconnecting with who you really are. The practice dissociates us—as sentient beings—from incessant mind activity. "You have to realize you've been locked in there with a maniac," writes Michael A. Singer in his best-selling book *The Untethered Soul*.[1] The maniac is your mind: the nonstop noise that feeds you an endless stream of negativity that you're not good enough, you're a failure, you're not making progress fast enough, you've slipped up one too many times, and that you'll never succeed. The mind can certainly be creative with its insults.

Meditation is not about turning those thoughts off, but rather, becoming the observer, or the watcher. Acknowledge that the voice is there and realize the stories it's spitting out aren't reality; they're just mind-made mental chatter. Choosing to disengage with the drama unfolding rather than getting wrapped up in it is what being mindfulness is all about. Eckhart Tolle, in *The Power of Now*, writes:

> One day you may catch yourself smiling at the voice in your head, as you would smile at the antics of a child. This means that you no longer take the content of your mind all that seriously, as your sense of self does not depend on it.[2]

Meditation helps you disassociate with the mind and not identify with your thoughts. This is the key to returning to our consciousness and "coming home," as Tara Brach writes, and experiencing inner calm and peace—a state we all strive for.[3]

MINDFUL TRAINING

Meditation is a long game and more akin to an ultramarathon than a sprint. One of the first steps is acknowledging that meditation isn't a means to an end but, rather, an ongoing, lifelong journey deep within ourselves. Here's the paradox: we can use our practice to set and achieve our goals, but meditation has no end goal or final destination. In one of our classes, Shifu Yuan Jing told me, "The practice is the goal in and of itself."

So how can meditation help us in our day-to-day fitness efforts? Becoming intensely present during athletic challenges and even during a training session at the gym can help us enjoy our workouts more. Further, surrendering to our circumstances or issues that arise during our workouts can help us better handle adversity. Instead of getting upset when someone is starting up on a machine you want to be using at the gym, let that energy you feel flow through you, and then go to another machine. When you surrender to what is, something interesting happens. You no longer resist and cause suffering and tension within yourself, but rather, your mind can now come up with creative solutions and even offer new ways to grow, like trying a new machine, which might end up being your new favorite.

In endurance sports like marathons and ultramarathons, the mental training is, in my opinion, even more important than the physical. My mindfulness practice: learning to be intensely present and surrendering to my circumstances helped me complete my first 100-mile endurance race. Not only did I finish, but I placed first in my gender category and third place overall. I'm not telling you this to brag. A lot went down in that race. I got lost, missed a loop, and had only a puny little dollar-store flashlight when the sun was going down. It poured rain with thunder and lightning for hours when I was running through the forest. If I had given in to my mind activity that was pure panic and anxiety, I would have quit at the next aid station and gotten a big DNF (did not finish). Instead, I surrendered and forced myself to accept what is (good or bad) and just let the race play out as it did. Everything worked out: My pacer met me at a different aid station with my drop bag that had the headlamp just before the sun came down. The race director graciously allowed me to do the loop I missed at the end of the race and let me have a complete finish.

It's not only in races, though. If we practice meditation, we can become more focused at the gym. A distracted or hyperactive mind—watching the clock, checking your text messages, going on social media while you train— will make the time pass slower. Being present, listening to your breathing, and feeling the sweat pouring down your face and the endorphins kick in is euphoric. Running through nature with beautiful scenery and piney smell is cathartic. When you meditate, you learn to heighten your senses around you. When your mind is still, you leave room to be fully engaged in the activity.

MINDFUL EATING

Mindful eating, or enjoying the sensations of our food, being fully present in the experience, is a way for us to eat less. In *Intuitive Eating*, the authors refer to this practice as getting in touch with our inner hunger signals. Eating slow, focusing on the taste of the food, taking slow bites, and feeling the sensations in our stomach may help us stop eating when we're full.[4] Many health professionals are now prescribing mindful eating as a method of retraining individuals with diabetes to change their eating behaviors.[5] In Jon Kabat-Zinn's best-selling book *Full Catastrophe Living*, he presents readers with the famous raisin challenge, summarized as follows:

Feel the texture and weight of the raisin, notice the smells, roll it between your fingers and notice how it feels on your fingertips, put it in your mouth (not yet chewing), but feeling the taste sensations, then chew slowly and notice the next sensations you feel, then when you finally swallow, reflect on the entire experience from beginning to end. You're engaging all your senses to be fully mindful as you interact with and consume the raisin.[6]

It's that "moment-by-moment" experience that we want to strive for, and to do that, we need to slow down. We don't need to eat every morsel of food like this (otherwise, we'd be sitting at the kitchen table for 10-plus hours per day), but trying to be fully present when you eat is a rewarding experience. Training ourselves to taste the food fully is a way not only to eat less but also to better enjoy the experience of eating—one of the many genuine pleasures and joys in life. Take time away from our work, away from our phones to just sit down and focus on the food, and the process of eating has a calming effect on our psyche; give it a try.

THE MENTAL GAME

To make any significant changes in our body, we know that we have to make changes with our mind. Observing the self-deprecating thoughts and removing ourselves can help us develop self-compassion. Training our mind takes work, time, and patience, and it's not an overnight kind of accomplishment. It's a lifelong commitment. But once you experience the inner calm, the quiet mind, and come to the realization that you are not your mind, you'll be able to much better deal with adversity, setbacks, and continue to learn, grow, and challenge yourself.

Conclusion

Well, here we are at the end of our journey together. I hope that this is just the start for you, and a start where you can find deep meaning in your training as I have. Looking inward and finding those *intrinsic* motivators is the key to a sustainable and enjoyable practice.

By building muscle and strength, I developed confidence, felt better, and had more energy to pursue bigger goals such as writing this book. I want you to experience the same personal success. As I mentioned earlier, I just hit my fourth year of consecutive running. If I felt like the effort was forced, there would be no way I'd be able to sustain my training day in and day out. Does that mean I want to run every day? No, not at all. I still have to push myself to overcome resistance and procrastination, just like everyone else. By adjusting my frames, however, and trying to extract the non-aesthetic or performance reasons why I run (to feel good, to give me energy, etc.), it's much easier to deal with the chatter in my head that would rather keep me stagnant and complacent.

I never wanted this book to be about some fad diet or unrealistic fitness plan. The truth is that there is no such thing as a universal diet or plan. Instead, I wanted to present information backed by science that's worked for me and others, in the hopes that you can take pieces of this information to apply to your fitness goals. You get to decide the role you want fitness to play in your life.

Remember that nothing is fixed. If you've struggled with body composition changes in the past (like I did) or following a training routine or nutrition plan, it doesn't mean that you're a failure or lack self-discipline, or even lazy. It just means that you may need to reframe *why* you train and the deeper meaning behind your goals. Until I took a course on creative productivity (called Amplify by Steve Pavlina), I struggled to work on this book. I was focused on the externals: the accolades, opening the doors to new opportunities, and other egocentric rewards. When I switched my focus to gaining competency in my research and writing abilities, and using the knowledge I've accumulated over the years to help others, I was able to achieve much more consistent creative flow.

I challenge you to do the same. I'll end with this reminder: remember that you're an explorer—a scientist. In your books, there's no such thing as failure. Each subsequent setback brings you closer to your own truth. *Finding* is about conducting life-long experiments, refining and tweaking as you go; it involves looking inward. *Your* is about taking ownership, being accountable and responsible for your own life. While we all come from different starting points and social locations—some born into privilege and some not—it's up to you to work with what you have and discover your own fitness and life journey, for yourself. As author Robert Greene purports, our chemical makeup and DNA will never be repeated in history; we are all truly unique.[1] Each of us has our own life purpose, our own unique *stride*. Your stride is not better or worse than anyone else's; it's simply yours. Understand that it's okay to not know what your stride is today. As you get older, things change; new interests emerge, while others you'll let go of. Your stride may change over time, and that's okay! Any nutrition and fitness plan will work for you if you *stick with it long enough*. It just takes time and patience. That's why you need to craft one that works for you, that makes you feel good, and all while supporting your *individualized* fitness goals. The more you show up, the more confidence you build, and the more you'll be able to deal with those pesky voices—setting you up for sustainable success over the long haul.

I genuinely hope this book helps you in some way. Now go *find your stride.*

Acknowledgments

I wouldn't have had the mental stamina to produce this book without the collaboration, support, and inspiration from so many other amazing people throughout the process. While writing is indeed an individualistic undertaking, the production of this book was very much a team effort.

First and foremost, I thank the entire team at Greenleaf Book Group that brought my rough manuscript draft to a finished and polished piece of art that I'm so proud of. A huge thank-you goes to my lead editor, Rebecca Logan, who oversaw the editorial process end-to-end to ensure cohesion; my developmental editor, Judy Marchman, who helped guide the book's flow and structure; my amazing copyeditors, Susan Flurry and Pam Nordberg, who ensured cohesive flow; my proofreader, Tonya Trybula; Jen Glynn, whose amazing project management skills kept us all organized and on schedule; the incredibly talented cover and book designer Mimi Bark; my distribution lead, Tiffany Barrientos; and my marketing lead, Amanda Marquette. I also thank Daniel Sandoval and Shannon Zuniga.

Next, I thank my amazing family, who have provided me with support and encouragement over the years, helping me build the confidence to pursue all my goals (despite how off the wall they may have been): my mom, Kate; my dad, Terry; my brother, Tom; my sister, Alex; and our family dog, Sadie (who gave me cuddles in the early morning, when I was in the process of writing the first, very rough draft). Special thanks go to my incredibly talented sister and best friend, Alex, who helped me along in this whole process, including assisting with my book submission to Greenleaf, offering pragmatic consultation on tough, content-related decisions, and even editing early pieces of my manuscript. I also thank my brilliant cousin Sara Ross, who has been a mentor and inspiration to me and who first introduced me to Greenleaf and helped me with the submission process.

I thank my best friend, Kayla Nezon, who's been a huge support system for me over the years and throughout this process and who gave me constructive criticism and insightful suggestions. I thank the amazing Sue Duffy for her creative input and aid in the launch of this book. I thank my good friend Kristian Kletke, who offered her insightful suggestions and unwavering support. Thanks also go to my good friend Kristie Holden, who helped me navigate the book-writing process from the outset.

Find Your Stride would not have been possible without the contribution and collaboration of other fitness professionals doing important work in the field. I thank Mike Rosa for his collaboration on this book and other creative projects. He is incredibly generous to share his wealth of knowledge in the fitness realm with others. I'm extremely grateful to Dr. Eric Helms, not only for his contribution to the field but also for reviewing an earlier draft of my manuscript, offering invaluable insights and constructive feedback on the training portion of the book. I also thank my friend Amber Cubitt, founder of Spoon In, for putting together delicious vegan nutrition plans for readers.

I am grateful to Chris Guillebeau, whose book *The Happiness of Pursuit* and invitation to the 2017 World Domination Summit changed my life. His ongoing inspiration and support over the last four years have meant the world to me. I also thank Steve Pavlina, whose course, Amplify, helped me develop the intrinsic motivation to endure on the hard days and show up consistently to my creative work. In addition, I thank Brad Stulberg and Steve Magness at the Growth Equation, who've taught me the principles and practices that made writing this book autotelic for me—they helped me enjoy the act of writing in and of itself.

Last, I thank the fitness experts whom I truly believe are spreading important messages and advice when it comes to fitness: Lauren Leavell, Shana Minei Spence, Meg Boggs, Ivy Felicia, Dalina Soto, Amanda Brooks, Michelle Segar, Stephanie Buttermore, Brad Schoenfeld, Jeff Nippard, Menno Henselmans, Paul Revelia, and Eric Trexler.

Resources

FURTHER READING

Books

The Art of Living by Thich Nhat Hanh

Can't Hurt Me by David Goggins

The Easy Way to Control Alcohol by Allen Carr

Eat and Run by Scott Jurek

Ego Is the Enemy by Ryan Holiday

Essays by Michel de Montaigne

Fearing the Black Body by Sabrina Strings

Finding Ultra by Rich Roll

Fitness for Every Body by Meg Boggs

The 5 Second Rule by Mel Robbins

Full Catastrophe Living by Jon Kabat-Zinn

The Happiness of Pursuit by Chris Guillebeau

Intuitive Eating by Elyse Resch and Evelyn Tribole

Man's Search for Meaning by Viktor E. Frankl

Mastery by Robert Greene

Mindset by Carol S. Dweck

No Sweat by Michelle Segar

The Passion Paradox by Brad Stulberg and Steve Magness

Peak Performance by Brad Stulberg and Steve Magness

The Power of Now by Eckhart Tolle

The Practice of Groundedness by Brad Stulberg

Radical Acceptance by Tara Brach

Think Again by Adam Grant

This Naked Mind by Annie Grace

The Untethered Soul by Michael A. Singer

Blogs

The Growth Equation: The Art, Science, and Practice of Success:
https://thegrowtheq.com/home

Eric Helms's *3D Muscle Journey*:
https://3dmusclejourney.com/about/eric-helms

Menno Henselmans's *Science to Master Your Physique*:
https://mennohenselmans.com

Ryan Holiday's *Meditations on Strategy and Life*:
https://ryanholiday.net/blog

Steve Pavlina's *Personal Development for Smart People*:
https://stevepavlina.com

YouTube Channels

Anabolic Aliens: https://www.youtube.com/user/AnabolicAliens

Stephanie Buttermore:
https://www.youtube.com/c/StephanieButtermore

Jeff Nippard: https://www.youtube.com/user/icecream4PRs

Paul Revelia:
https://www.youtube.com/channel/UCykSWsfEKRES6RDotQF6ChQ

Will Tennyson:
https://www.youtube.com/channel/UCB2wtYpfbCpYDc5TeTwuqFA

MEAL PLANS

Five-Day Meal Plan (About 2,000 Calories, > 145 g Protein Daily)

	Meal	Carbohy-drates	Fats	Protein	Calories
MONDAY					
Breakfast	**Scrambled eggs** • 1 whole egg and 1/2 cup egg whites • mixed veggies: red and green pepper, mushrooms • 1 oz. cheddar cheese • topped with 1/4 cup salsa	20	14	33	345
Snack	• Quest chocolate chip cookie dough protein bar • medium apple	30	9	21	295
Lunch	**Open-faced sandwich on rice cakes** • 2 Quaker Crispy Minis tomato and basil rice cakes • 1/2 medium avocado • 4 oz. grilled chicken breast seasoned with roasted garlic and pepper seasoning	69	18	73	362
Snack	• 12 raw almonds • 7 cups Skinny Pop popcorn (2 servings) • 1 tbsp. spirulina powder (mixed with water and 1 packet stevia)	33	27	11	408
Dinner	**Turkey burgers** • 4 oz. lean ground turkey • 100 g sweet potato fries • 1 tbsp, olive oil • 1 cup roasted Brussels sprouts	29	21	26	403
Snack	• 3/4 cup plain Greek yogurt mixed with no-sugar Jell-O chocolate pudding cup	20	1	19	170
Total		201	90	183	1,983

continued

TUESDAY					
Breakfast	**Protein pancakes** • 1 mashed banana • 1 scoop Vega protein and greens • 1/4 cup liquid egg whites • 1 tbsp. unsweetened almond milk • topped with 3 tablespoons no-sugar-added maple syrup	40	2	28	285
Snack	• 1/4 cup hummus • 3 oz. snap peas • 3 oz. baby carrots • 1 scoop whey isolate protein mixed • 1 cup almond milk	26	16	34	372
Lunch	**Tempeh wrap** • 1 whole-wheat wrap • 100 g grilled tempeh • cucumber, lettuce, tomato • 2 tbsp. light mayo	37	21	23	417
Snack	• Quest chocolate chip cookie dough protein bar • medium apple	30	9	21	295
Dinner	• 4 oz. grilled flank steak • 100 g roasted yellow potatoes • roasted asparagus • 1 tbsp. olive oil	20	22	28	396
Snack	• 3/4 cup Greek yogurt • 1/2 cup mixed berries • 1 packet stevia • 12 raw almonds • 1/2 pear	44	7	21	283
Total		197	77	155	2,048

WEDNESDAY					
Breakfast	**Tofu scramble** • 85 g tofu • red and green pepper, mushrooms • 1/4 Daiya vegan cheddar cheese • 1/4 cup salsa	28	10	14	264
Snack	**Protein shake** • 1.5 scoops whey isolate protein powder blended with 2 cups almond milk and ice	5	10	41	253
Lunch	• 1 cup lamb vindaloo • mixed green salad • 4 tbsp. balsamic vinegar • 1 tsp. olive oil	40	19	26	440
Snack	• 7 cups Skinny Pop popcorn (2 servings)	30	20	4	300
Dinner	**Chicken fried rice** • 4 oz. chicken • 1 cup cooked brown rice • 1.5 cups baby bok choy • 1 cup broccoli • 1 egg • 1 tbsp. hoisin • 1 tbsp. soy sauce • 1 tbsp. sriracha	50	12	41	479
Snack	• 3/4 cup Greek yogurt • 1/2 cup mixed berries • 1 packet stevia • 12 raw almonds • 1/2 pear	44	7	21	283
Total		197	78	147	2,019

continued

THURSDAY					
Breakfast	**Poached eggs on rice cakes** • 2 full poached eggs • 1/2 avocado • 2 Quaker Crispy Minis gluten-free white cheddar rice cakes	23	21	16	353
Snack	**Protein shake** • 1.5 scoops whey isolate protein powder blended with 2 cups almond milk and ice	5	10	41	253
Lunch	**Tempeh sandwich** • 2 slices whole-wheat bread (toasted) • 100 g tempeh • 1 cup arugula • 1 oz. sun-dried tomatoes • 1/2 avocado (mixed with lemon and finely chopped onion) • seasoned with salt and pepper	67	24	31	577
Snack	• Quest chocolate chip cookie dough protein bar • medium apple	30	9	21	295
Dinner	• 1.5 cups homemade sweet potato shepherd's pie (with ground turkey) • 2 cups steamed broccoli	46	6	21	312
Snack	• 1 cup cottage cheese • 1 cup chopped mango	38	3	31	299
Total		209	73	161	2,089

FRIDAY					
Breakfast	**Scrambled eggs** • 1 whole egg and 1/2 cup egg whites • mixed veggies: red and green pepper, mushrooms • 1 oz. cheddar cheese • topped with 1/4 cup salsa	20	14	33	345
Snack	• 1 protein bar birthday cake flavor • 2 tbsp. spirulina mixed with water	25	8	28	270
Lunch	**Turkey burgers** • 4 oz. lean ground turkey • 1 cup steamed broccoli • 1 cup sautéed kale with garlic • 1 tsp. olive oil	12	13	27	264
Snack	• 1/2 cup cottage cheese • 12 almonds	9	8	18	183
Dinner	**Pita pizzas** • 1 whole-wheat pita • 2 oz. mozzarella cheese • mushrooms and green pepper • 30 g pepperoni	36	24	25	458
Snack	• 1 tub Halo Top cookie dough ice cream topped with 3/4 cup Reese's Puffs cereal	92	14	21	500
Total		194	81	152	2,020

Five-Day Meal Plan (About 2,800–3,000 Calories, > 175 g Protein Daily)

	Meal	Macros (g)			
		Carbohy-drates	Fats	Protein	Calories
MONDAY					
Breakfast	**Scrambled eggs and avocado toast** • 3 whole eggs • 1/2 cup egg whites • red and green pepper, mushrooms • 2 oz. cheddar cheese • 1/4 cup salsa • 1 slice whole-wheat toast • 1/2 avocado	39	46	58	790
Snack	• Quest chocolate chip cookie dough protein bar • medium apple	30	9	21	295
Lunch	**PB banana wrap** • 1 whole-wheat wrap • 2 tbsp. peanut butter • 1 whole banana • 1 scoop whey isolate protein (mixed with 2 cups almond milk)	65	25	46	655
Snack	• 1 tbsp. spirulina powder (mixed with water and 1 pack stevia) • 1/4 cup hummus • 1 cup snap peas • 1 cup baby carrots • 1 serving Skinny Pop popcorn (3 3/4 cup)	43	20	13	407
Dinner	• 4 oz. grilled salmon • 100 g sweet potato • grilled asparagus • 1 tbsp. olive oil	31	28	41	525
Snack	• 3/4 cup Greek yogurt • 1/2 cup mixed berries • 1 packet stevia • 12 raw almonds • 1/2 pear	44	7	21	283
Total		252	135	200	2,955

TUESDAY					
Breakfast	**PB banana wrap** • 1 whole-wheat wrap • 2 tbsp. peanut butter • 1 whole banana • 1 scoop whey isolate protein (mixed with 2 cups almond milk)	65	25	46	655
Snack	• Quest chocolate chip cookie dough protein bar • medium apple	30	9	21	295
Lunch	**Chicken club sandwich** • 4 oz chicken breast • 2 slices bacon • 1/2 avocado • tomato • 2 tbsp. light mayo • 2 slices whole-wheat toast	51	32	40	637
Snack	• 1/4 cup hummus • 3 oz. snap peas • 3 oz. baby carrots • 1 scoop whey isolate protein mixed with 1 cup almond milk	26	16	34	372
Dinner	**Chicken fried rice** • 4 oz. chicken • 1 cup cooked brown rice • 1.5 cups baby bok choy • 1 cup broccoli • 1 egg • 1 tbsp. hoisin • 1 tbsp. soy sauce • 1 tbsp. sriracha	50	12	41	479
Snack	• 3/4 cup Greek yogurt • 1/2 cup mixed berries • 1 packet stevia • 12 raw almonds • 1/2 pear • 1 tbsp. peanut butter • 3/4 cup Chex cinnamon cereal	72	16	26	493
Total		294	110	208	2,931

continued

WEDNESDAY

Breakfast	**Protein oats** • 1 cup oatmeal (dry) • 1 scoop whey isolate protein powder • 1 banana • 12 almonds • 1 cup almond milk	85	16	44	644
Snack	• 1 protein bar, birthday cake flavor • medium apple	36	8	20	270
Lunch	**Tempeh sandwich** • 2 slices whole-wheat bread (toasted) • 200 g tempeh • 1 cup arugula • 1 oz. sun-dried tomatoes • 1/2 avocado (mixed with lemon and finely chopped onion) • seasoned with salt and pepper	92	30	50	727
Snack	• 3/4 cup Greek yogurt • 1/2 cup mixed berries • 1 packet stevia • 12 raw almonds • 1/2 pear	44	7	21	283
Dinner	• 4 oz grilled flank steak • 100 g roasted yellow potatoes • roasted asparagus • 1 tbsp. olive oil	20	22	28	396
Snack	• 1 tub Halo Top cookie dough ice cream topped with 3/4 cup Reese's Puffs cereal	92	14	21	500
Total		369	97	184	2,820

THURSDAY					
Breakfast	**PB banana wrap** • 1 whole-wheat wrap • 2 tbsp. peanut butter • 1 whole banana • 1 scoop whey isolate protein (mixed with 2 cups almond milk)	65	25	46	655
Snack	• 1 protein, bar birthday cake flavor • medium apple	36	8	20	270
Lunch	**Tempeh wrap** • 1 whole-wheat wrap • 100 g grilled tempeh • cucumber, lettuce, tomato • 2 tbsp. light mayo	37	21	23	417
Snack	• 1/4 cup hummus • 3 oz. snap peas • 3 oz. baby carrots • 1 scoop whey isolate protein mixed • 1 cup almond milk	26	16	34	372
Dinner	**Tuna poke bowl** • 3–4 oz sushi-grade tuna • 1/2 cup white or brown rice • 1/2 avocado • 1/2 cup chopped cucumbers • 1/4 cup edamame • 1/4 cup sliced radish • tbsp scallions • 1 tsp sesame seeds • 1 tsp grated ginger • 2 tsp rice wine vinegar • 1 tsp soy sauce • 1 tsp sesame oil	79	39	34	590
Snack	• 3/4 cup Greek yogurt • 1/2 cup mixed berries • 1 packet stevia • 12 raw almonds • 1/2 pear • 1 tbsp. peanut butter • 3/4 cup Chex cinnamon cereal	72	16	26	493
Total		315	125	183	2,797

continued

FRIDAY					
Breakfast	**Scrambled eggs** • 1 whole egg and 1/2 cup egg whites • mixed veggies: red and green pepper, mushrooms • 1 oz. cheddar cheese • topped with 1/4 cup salsa	20	14	33	345
Snack	• 1 protein bar, birthday cake flavor • medium apple	36	8	20	270
Lunch	• 1 cup lamb vindaloo • mixed green salad • 4 tbsp. balsamic vinegar • 1 tsp. olive oil	40	19	26	440
Snack	• 12 raw almonds • 7 cups Skinny Pop popcorn (2 servings) • Protein shake: 1.5 scoops whey isolate protein powder blended with 2 cups almond milk and ice	38	37	52	661
Dinner	**Pita Pizzas** • 2 whole-wheat pitas • 4 oz. mozzarella cheese • 2 cup mushrooms • green pepper • 60 g pepperoni	72	48	50	916
Snack	• 1 tub Halo Top cookie dough ice cream topped with 3/4 cup Reese's Puffs cereal	92	14	21	500
Total		298	140	202	3,132

Five-Day Vegan Meal Plan (2,000–2,300 Calories, 145–175 g Protein Daily)

		Macros (g)			
	Meal	Carbohy-drates	Fats	Protein	Calories
MONDAY					
Breakfast	**Green smoothie** • 1/4 banana • 1 cup spinach • 1.5 scoop vegan protein powder (30 g) • 1 cup soy milk • 3 tbsp. hemp hearts • 3 ice cubes	21	20	48	461
Snack	• Vega protein bar	27	10	20	290
Lunch	**Sweet balsamic salad** • 3/4 cup black beans • 1 cup cucumber, chopped • 1/2 cup cherry tomatoes, halved • 1 cup kale, chopped • 1 serving chickpea pasta (2 oz.) • 1/3 cup tempeh • 1/4 cup fresh parsley, chopped • pinch salt and pepper • sweet balsamic dressing • 1 tbsp. Dijon mustard • 1 tbsp. tahini • 1 tbsp. balsamic vinegar • 1/4 tbsp. maple syrup	96	18	44	711
Snack	**Chia pudding** • 1 cup almond milk • 4 tbsp. chia seeds • 1 tbsp. vanilla • 1/2 grapefruit, peeled and sliced —Let sit in refrigerator for 1–2 hours.	35	15	14	329

continued

Dinner	**Sweet lentil curry**
	• 1 tsp. coconut oil
	• 1/4 cup onion, diced
	• 1/2 tbsp. garlic, minced
	• 1/2 tbsp. curry powder
	  —Sauté until onions are
	   translucent.
	• 1/2 cup firm tofu, cubed
	  —Let tofu sear until browned
	• 1/4 cup red lentils
	• 1 cup broccoli florets
	• 1/4 cup coconut milk
	• 1 cup water
	• 1 tbsp. agave syrup
	• 1 tsp. salt
	• 1/4 cup frozen peas
	  —Stir and cover. Let simmer on
	   medium-low heat for 30–40
	   minutes.
		68	17	25	493

Total		247	80	151	2,284

TUESDAY

Breakfast	**Grapefruit parfait** • 1 grapefruit, peeled and sliced • 3/4 cup Silk vanilla almond yogurt • 2 tbsp. chia seeds • 2 tbsp. hemp hearts • 1.75 scoop vegan protein powder (35 g)	59	31	54	714
Snack	• Vega protein bar	27	10	20	290
Lunch	**Avocado toast** • 1 serving Mestemacher protein bread (see package) • 1/2 avocado, mashed • 4 slices tomato • 120 g seared tempeh • 1 tsp. chili flakes	37	25	36	509

Dinner	**Falafel bowl**	95	14	36	622
	• 1 tbsp. tahini				
	• 1/4 cup onion, diced				
	• 1/2 tbsp. garlic, minced				
	• 1/3 cup chickpeas, rinsed				
	• 2/3 cup black beans, rinsed				
	• 1 tbsp. lemon juice				
	• 1/8 cup fresh cilantro, chopped				
	• 1/2 tbsp. salt				
	• 1/2 tbsp. cumin				
	• 2 tbsp. chickpea flour				
	• 1/2 tbsp. paprika				
	• 1 tsp. basil				
	—Use food processor to blend until a doughy consistency has formed. Roll into balls and place on a nonstick baking sheet. Bake at 350°F for 40 minutes.				
	• 1 cup mushroom				
	• 15 spears asparagus				
	—Roast vegetables on a nonstick baking sheet for 20 minutes.				
	• 2 cups romaine lettuce, chopped for bowl's base				
Total		218	80	146	2,135
WEDNESDAY					
Breakfast	**Tofu scramble**	33	34	35	547
	• 1/2 tbsp. olive oil				
	• 1/8 cup onion, diced				
	• 1/2 tbsp. garlic, minced				
	• 1 cup firm tofu, crumbled				
	• 1 tbsp. chili powder				
	• pinch salt and pepper				
	• 1 cup green bell pepper, diced				
	• —Cook on medium heat for 10–15 minutes, stirring occasionally.				
	• 1 cup spinach				
	• —Add spinach and cook for another 3 minutes.				
	• 1/2 avocado, sliced				
	• 1 serving Mestemacher protein bread (see package)				

continued

Snack	**Super peanut butter protein shake** • 1 cup soy milk • 1.5 scoop vegan protein powder (30 g) • 3 tbsp. PB2 peanut butter powder • 1/4 banana • 3 ice cubes	24	9	46	361
Lunch	**Mexican heat salad** • 3/4 cup black beans • 1/8 cup corn • 1/8 cup red onion, diced • 1/8 cup black olives, sliced • 1/2 cup bell pepper, diced • 1 jalapeño, diced (without seeds) • 1/2 cup edamame • 1 cup cherry tomatoes, halved • 1/8 cup fresh cilantro, chopped • 2 cups romaine, chopped **Hot heat dressing** • 1 tbsp. olive oil • 2 tbsp. lemon juice • 1 tsp. chili flakes • 1 tsp. chili powder • pinch salt and pepper	62	25	22	558

Dinner	**Zucchini noodle pesto pasta**
	• 120 g seared tempeh
	• 1 zucchini, spiralized
	  —Simmer tempeh for 5 minutes and drain excess water. Toss zucchini in pan and cook on medium heat for 5 minutes.
	
	Pesto
	• 1/2 avocado
	• 1/4 cup soaked cashews (2–4 hrs.)
	• 3 tbsp. nutritional yeast
	• 1/2 tsp. salt
	• 1/2 tsp. pepper
	  —Blend all ingredients in a food processor, adding water as needed. Add pesto to noodles and simmer for 1–2 minutes.
		40	33	42	604

Total		159	101	145	2,070

THURSDAY					
Breakfast	**Nuts and berry smoothie** • 1/4 banana • 1/2 cup frozen mixed berries • 1.5 scoops protein powder • 1 cup soy milk • 1 tbsp. almond butter • 3 ice cubes	28	16	41	401
Snack	• Vega protein bar	27	10	20	290
Lunch	**Thai summer slaw** • 1 cup red cabbage, chopped finely • 1/4 cup parsley, chopped • 3/4 cup chickpeas • 2 tbsp. sesame seeds **Slaw dressing** • 1 tbsp. soy sauce • 1 tbsp. peanut butter • 1 tbsp. maple syrup • 1/2 tbsp. olive oil	56	26	18	506
Snack	**Chia pudding** • 1 cup almond milk • 4 tbsp. chia seeds • 1 tsp. vanilla • 1/2 grapefruit, peeled and sliced —Let sit in refrigerator for 1–2 hours.	35	15	14	329

continued

Dinner	**TVP Bolognese**
	
	• 1/2 cup TVP (textured vegetable protein)
	  —Simmer TVP in a frying pan for 5 minutes.
	• 1/8 cup onion, diced
	• 1/2 tbsp. garlic
	• pinch salt and pepper
	• 2 fresh tomatoes, chopped
	• 1 tbsp. basil
	• 1 cup broccoli florets
	  —Add ingredients to pan and sauté for 10 minutes.
	• 3 oz. The Only Bean Edamame Pasta
	  —Cook pasta as instructed and combine with sauce.
		57	8	63	508

Total		203	75	156	2,034
FRIDAY					
Breakfast	**Overnight chilled oats** • 1 tsp. vanilla extract • 1/4 cup quick oats • 1 scoop vegan protein powder (20 g) • 1 cup soy milk • 1 tbsp. chia seeds • 1 tbsp. pepita seed butter • 1/2 cup mixed berries —Mix all ingredients in a bowl and leave in the fridge overnight.	79	18	43	657
Snack	• Vega protein bar	27	10	20	290

Lunch	**Roasted veggies and hummus** • 1 cup zucchini, sliced • 1 cup eggplant, sliced • 1 tbsp. olive oil • 120 g tempeh • pinch salt and pepper —Coat vegetables in oil and sprinkle with seasoning. Bake vegetables and tempeh for 30 minutes at 350°F. • 1/4 cup hummus • 1 cup cucumber, sliced • 1/8 cup cashews	36	40	34	630

Dinner	**Mexican lettuce wraps**
	 • 3/4 cup TVP
	 • 1/3 cup black beans
	 • 1/8 cup red onion, diced
	 • 1 tbsp. chili powder
	 • 1 tsp. cumin
	 • 1/2 tsp. pepper
	 • 1 cup spinach
	   —Add ingredients to a pan with 1/2 cup water and cover. Cook over medium heat for 15 minutes, stirring occasionally.
	 • 5 romaine lettuce leaves
	 • 1/2 avocado, sliced
	 • 1/2 tomato, sliced
	   —Add all ingredients into romaine leaves.
		81	13	54	648

Total		223	81	151	2,225

Five-Day Vegan Meal Plan (2,800–3,250 Calories, 200+ g Protein Daily)

	Meal	Macros (g)			
		Carbohy-drates	Fats	Protein	Calories
MONDAY					
Breakfast	**Green smoothie** • 1/2 banana • 2 cups spinach • 2 scoops protein powder (40 g) • 1 cup soy milk • 3 tbsp. hemp hearts • 3 ice cubes • 1 tbsp. peanut butter	35	30	63	644
Snack	• Vega protein bar • 1/4 cup almonds	35	28	28	497
Lunch	**Sweet balsamic salad** • 3/4 cup black beans • 1 cup cucumber, chopped • 1/2 cup cherry tomatoes, halved • 1 cup kale, chopped • 1 serving chickpea pasta (2 oz.) • 1/3 cup tempeh • 1/4 cup parsley, chopped • pinch salt and pepper **Sweet balsamic dressing** • 1 tbsp. Dijon mustard • 1 tbsp. tahini • 1 tbsp. balsamic vinegar • 1/4 tbsp. maple syrup	96	18	44	711
Snack	**Chia pudding** • 1 cup almond milk • 4 tbsp. chia seeds • 1 tsp. vanilla • 1/2 grapefruit, peeled and sliced —Let sit in refrigerator for 1–2 hours. • 2 squares Mid-Day Squares chocolate	53	37	26	639

Dinner	**Sweet lentil curry**
	• 1 tsp. coconut oil
	• 1/4 cup onion, diced
	• 1/2 tbsp. garlic, minced
	• 1/2 tbsp. curry powder
	  —Sauté until onions are
	    translucent.
	• 3/4 cup firm tofu, cubed
	  —Let tofu sear until browned.
	• 1/2 cup red lentils
	• 1/4 cup sweet potato
	• 1 cup broccoli florets
	• 1/4 cup coconut milk
	• 2 cups water
	• 1 tbsp. agave syrup
	• 1 tsp. salt
	• 1/4 cup frozen peas
	  —Stir and cover. Let simmer on
	    medium-low heat for 30–40
	    minutes.
		107	21	43	753

Total		326	134	204	3,244

TUESDAY

Breakfast	**Grapefruit parfait** • 1 grapefruit, peeled and sliced • 3/4 cup Silk vanilla almond yogurt • 2 tbsp. chia seeds • 2 tbsp. hemp hearts • 1.75 scoop vegan protein powder (35 g)	59	31	54	714
Snack	• 1 Vega protein bar • 1/4 cup pepita seeds • 1/4 cup raspberries	35	25	29	478
Lunch	**Avocado toast** • 1 serving Mestemacher protein bread (see package) • 1/2 avocado, mashed • 4 slices tomato • 120 g seared tempeh • 1 tsp. chili flakes	37	25	36	509

continued

Snack	**Edamame pasta salad** • 3 oz. The Only Bean Edamame Pasta • 1/2 tbsp. sesame oil • 1/4 cup red bell pepper, chopped • 1 tbsp. soy sauce • 2 tsp. maple syrup • 2 cups spinach, chopped • 1/4 cup slivered almonds	36	37	48	656
Dinner	**Falafel bowl** • 1 tbsp. tahini • 1/4 cup onion, diced • 1/2 tbsp. garlic, minced • 1/3 cup chickpeas, rinsed • 2/3 cup black beans, rinsed • 1 tbsp. lemon juice • 1/8 cup fresh cilantro, chopped • 1/2 tsp. salt • 1/2 tbsp. cumin • 2 tbsp. chickpea flour • 1/2 tsp. paprika • 1 tsp. basil —Use a food processor to blend until a doughy consistency has formed. Roll into balls and place on nonstick baking sheet. Bake at 350°F for 40 minutes. • 1 cup mushrooms • 15 spears asparagus —Roast vegetables on a nonstick baking sheet for 20 minutes. • 2 cups romaine lettuce, chopped for bowl's base	95	14	36	622
Total		262	132	203	2,979

WEDNESDAY					
Breakfast	**Tofu scramble** • 1/2 tbsp. olive oil • 1/8 cup onion diced • 1/2 tbsp. minced garlic • 1 cup firm tofu, crumbled • 1 tbsp. chili powder • pinch salt and pepper • 1 cup green bell pepper, diced —Cook on medium heat for 10–15 minutes, stirring occasionally. • 1 cup spinach —Add spinach and cook for another 3 minutes. • 1/2 avocado, sliced • 1 serving Mestemacher protein bread (see package)	33	34	35	547
Snack	**Super peanut butter protein shake** • 1 cup soy milk • 1.5 scoop vegan protein powder (30 g) • 3 tbsp. PB2 peanut butter powder • 1/4 banana • 3 ice cubes • Iron Vegan protein bar	53	18	62	591
Lunch	**Mexican heat salad** • 3/4 cup black beans • 1/8 cup corn • 1/8 cup red onion, diced • 1/8 cup black olives, sliced • 1/2 cup bell pepper, diced • 1 jalapeño, diced (without seeds) • 1/2 cup edamame • 1 cup cherry tomatoes, halved • 1/8 cup fresh cilantro, chopped • 2 cups romaine, chopped **Hot heat dressing** • 1 tbsp. olive oil • 2 tbsp. lemon juice • 1 tsp. chili flakes • 1 tsp. chili powder • pinch salt and pepper	70	36	49	798

continued

Snack	**Vegan snack plate** • 1/2 apple sliced • 2 tbsp. pumpkin seed butter • 1 cup celery sticks • 1/4 cup hummus • 1 packet Noble Jerky vegan jerky	60	27	28	567
Dinner	**Zucchini noodle pesto pasta** • 120 g seared tempeh • 1 zucchini spiralized —Simmer tempeh for 5 minutes and drain excess water. Toss zucchini in pan and cook on medium heat for 5 minutes. **Pesto** • 1/2 avocado • 1/4 cup soaked cashews (2–4 hrs.) • 3 tbsp. nutritional yeast • 1/2 tsp. salt • 1/2 tsp. pepper —Blend all ingredients in a food processor, adding water as needed. Add pesto to noodles and simmer 1–2 minutes.	40	33	42	604
Total		256	148	216	3,107
THURSDAY					
Breakfast	**Nuts and berry smoothie** • 1/4 banana • 1/2 cup frozen mixed berries • 1.5 scoops protein powder • 1 cup soy milk • 1 tbsp. almond butter • 3 ice cubes	37	25	48	550
Snack	• Vega protein bar • 1 cup carrot, sliced • 1 cup cucumber, sliced • 1/4 cup hummus	47	16	24	428

Lunch	**Thai summer slaw** • 1 cup red cabbage, chopped finely • 1/4 cup parsley, chopped • 3/4 cup chickpeas • 2 tbsp. sesame seeds **Slaw dressing** • 1 tbsp. soy sauce • 1 tbsp. peanut butter • 1 tbsp. maple syrup • 1/2 tbsp. olive oil	111	32	30	819

Snack	**Chia pudding**
	• 1 cup almond milk
	• 4 tbsp. chia seeds
	• 1 tsp. vanilla
	• 1/2 grapefruit, peeled and sliced
	  —Let sit in refrigerator 1–2 hours.
	• 2 squares Mid-Day Squares
	  chocolate
		57	43	26	709

Dinner	**TVP Bolognese**
	• 1/2 cup TVP (textured vegetable protein)
	  —Simmer TVP in a frying pan for 5 minutes.
	• 1/8 cup diced onion
	• 1/2 tbsp. garlic
	• pinch salt and pepper
	• 2 fresh tomatoes, chopped
	• 1 tbsp. basil
	• 1 cup broccoli florets
	  —Add ingredients to pan and sauté 10 minutes.
	• 3 oz. The Only Bean Edamame Pasta
	  —Cook pasta as instructed and combine with sauce.
		64	8	75	588

Total		316	124	203	3,094

continued

FRIDAY					
Breakfast	**Overnight chilled oats** • 1 tsp. vanilla extract • 1/4 cup quick oats • 1 scoop vegan protein powder (20 g) • 1 cup soy milk • 1 tbsp. chia seeds • 1 tbsp. pepita seed butter • 1/2 cup mixed berries —Mix all ingredients in a bowl and leave in the fridge overnight.	79	18	43	657
Snack	• Vega protein bar • apple	49	10	20	370
Lunch	**Roasted veggies and hummus** • 1 cup zucchini, sliced • 1 cup eggplant, sliced • 1 tbsp. olive oil • 120 g tempeh • pinch salt and pepper —Coat vegetables in oil and sprinkle with seasoning. Bake vegetables and tempeh 30 minutes at 350°F. • 1/4 cup hummus • 1 cup cucumber, sliced • 1/8 cup cashews	36	40	34	630
Snack	**Seitan sandwich** • 1 serving Mestemacher protein bread (see package) • 2 servings (160 g) Gusta vegan seitan sliced • 2 tbsp. tofu dip	26	25	50	522

Dinner	**Mexican lettuce wraps**	81	13	54	648
	• 3/4 cup TVP (textured vegetable protein)				
	• 1/3 cup black beans				
	• 1/8 cup red onion, diced				
	• 1 tbsp. chili powder				
	• 1 tsp. cumin				
	• 1/2 tsp. pepper				
	• 1 cup spinach —Add ingredients to a pan with 1/2 cup water and cover. Cook over medium heat 15 minutes, stirring occasionally.				
	• 5 romaine lettuce leaves				
	• 1/2 avocado, sliced				
	• 1/2 tomato, sliced —Add all ingredients into romaine leaves.				
Total		271	106	201	2827

TRAINING PLANS

Push/Pull/Legs (Six Days a Week)

Monday: push workout—chest, triceps, and front and side delts

Exercise 1: Barbell bench press (5 sets, 5 reps)1

Exercise 2: Barbell decline bench press (4 sets, 6 reps)

Exercise 3: Dumbbell incline fly (3 sets, 8 reps)

Exercise 4: Machine fly (3 sets, 10 reps)

Exercise 5: Barbell kneeling landmine shoulder press (3 sets, 8 reps)

Exercise 6: Neutral-grip shoulder press machine (3 sets, 10 reps)

Exercise 7: Lateral raise machine (3 sets, 12 reps)

Exercise 8: Dumbbell close-grip bench press (3 sets, 12 reps)

Exercise 9: Cable bar pushdown (3 sets, 15 reps)

Volume: 30 sets

Tuesday: pull workout—back, rear delts, biceps, and forearms

Exercise 1: Barbell bent-over overhand row (5 sets, 5 reps)

Exercise 2: Supinated lat pulldown (4 sets, 6 reps)

Exercise 3: Cable close-grip seated low row (3 sets, 8 reps)

Exercise 4: Cable one-arm underhand row (3 sets, 10 reps)

Exercise 5: Dumbbell shrug (3 sets, 12 reps)

Exercise 6: Dumbbell reverse fly (3 sets, 8 reps)

Exercise 7: Cable face pull (3 sets, 10 reps)

Exercise 8: Cable curl (3 sets, 12 reps)

Exercise 9: Dumbbell alternating hammer curl (3 sets, 15 reps)

Volume: 30 sets

Wednesday: legs and core

Exercise 1: Barbell back squat (5 sets, 5 reps)

Exercise 2: Barbell alternating forward lunge (4 sets, 6 reps)

Exercise 3: Dumbbell straight-legged dead lift (4 sets, 8 reps)

Exercise 4: Leg extension machine (4 sets, 10 reps)

Exercise 5: Glute pushback machine (3 sets, 12 reps)

Exercise 6: Hip adduction machine (3 sets, 15 reps)

Exercise 7: Calf raise machine (4 sets, 15 reps)

Exercise 8: Captain chair leg raises (3 sets, 15 reps)

Volume: 30 sets

Tabata HIIT: 20/10 intervals for four-minute circuit:

Exercise 1: Bikes

Exercise 2: Leg raises

Exercise 3: Penguins

Exercise 4: Toe touches

Thursday: chest, triceps, and front and side delts

Exercise 1: Barbell overhead press (5 sets, 5 reps)

Exercise 2: Dumbbell seated alternating front raise (4 sets, 6 reps)

Exercise 3: Cable one-arm side raise (3 sets, 8 reps)

Exercise 4: Dumbbell seated Arnold press (3 sets, 10 reps)

Exercise 5: Dumbbell incline bench press (3 sets, 8 reps)

Exercise 6: Cable downward chest fly (3 sets, 10 reps)

Exercise 7: Neutral grip chest press machine (3 sets, 12 reps)

Exercise 8: EZ bar overhead extension (3 sets, 12 reps)

Exercise 9: EZ bar skull crusher (3 sets, 15 reps)

Volume: 30 sets

Friday: back, rear delts, biceps, and forearms

Exercise 1: Barbell bent-over underhand row (5 sets, 5 reps)

Exercise 2: Wide-grip lat pulldown (4 sets, 6 reps)

Exercise 3: Straight-arm pulldown (3 sets, 8 reps)

Exercise 4: Dumbbell one-arm row (3 sets, 10 reps)

Exercise 5: Cable bar close-grip upright row (3 sets, 12 reps)

Exercise 6: Cable standing reverse fly (3 sets, 8 reps)

Exercise 7: Machine reverse fly (3 sets, 10 reps)

Exercise 8: Dumbbell supinated curl (3 sets, 12 reps)

Exercise 9: EZ bar reverse grip curl (3 sets, 15 reps)

Volume: 30 sets

Saturday: legs and core

Exercise 1: Leg press (5 sets, 5 reps)

Exercise 2: Leg press calf extensions (3 sets, 30 reps)

Exercise 3: Dumbbell Bulgarian split squat (4 sets, 6 reps)

Exercise 4: Barbell Romanian dead lift (4 sets, 8 reps)

Exercise 5: Cable pull-through (3 sets, 10 reps)

Exercise 6: Lying leg curl machine (3 sets, 12 reps)

Exercise 7: Hip abduction machine (3 sets, 15 reps)

Exercise 8: Kneeling cable crunch (3 sets, 15 reps)

Volume: 28 sets

Tabata HIIT: *20/10 intervals for four-minute circuit:*

Exercise 1: Russian twists

Exercise 2: Reverse crunch

Exercise 3: Starfish

Exercise 4: Speed crunches

Upper/Lower (Six Days a Week)

Monday: upper body

Exercise 1: Barbell standing overhead press (4 sets, 6 reps)

Exercise 2: Barbell incline bench press (3 sets, 8 reps)

Exercise 3: Cable close-grip seated low row (3 sets, 8 reps)

Exercise 4: Machine reverse fly (3 sets, 8 reps)

Exercise 5: Compound set: dumbbell side raise and dumbbell front raise (3 sets, 10 reps)

Exercise 6: Compound set: dumbbell fly and dumbbell bench press (3 sets, 10 reps)

Exercise 7: Dumbbell close-grip bench press (3 sets, 8 reps)

Exercise 8: Dumbbell supinated curl (3 sets, 8 reps)

Exercise 9: Superset: dumbbell skull crusher and dumbbell hammer curl (3 sets, 10 reps)

Exercise 10: Kneeling cable crunch (4 sets, 12 reps)

Volume: *32 sets*

Tuesday: lower body

Exercise 1: Barbell back squat (5 sets, 5 reps)

Exercise 2: Barbell alternating forward lunge (4 sets, 6 reps)

Exercise 3: Dumbbell straight-legged dead lift (4 sets, 8 reps)

Exercise 4: Leg extension machine (3 sets, 10 reps)

Exercise 5: Glute pushback machine (3 sets, 12 reps)

Exercise 6: Hip adduction machine (3 sets, 15 reps)

Exercise 7: Calf raise machine (4 sets, 15 reps)

Volume: *26 sets*

Wednesday: upper body

Exercise 1: Barbell bench press (4 sets, 6 reps)

Exercise 2: Supinated lat pulldown (3 sets, 8 reps)

Exercise 3: Dumbbell seated shoulder press (3 sets, 8 reps)

Exercise 4: Dumbbell reverse fly (3 sets, 8 reps)

Exercise 5: Compound set: cable downward chest fly and plate Svend press (3 sets, 10 reps)

Exercise 6: Compound set: barbell one-arm landmine row and barbell T-row (3 sets, 10 reps)

Exercise 7: Cable bar pushdown (3 sets, 8 reps)

Exercise 8: Cable bar curl (3 sets, 8 reps)

Exercise 9: Superset: EZ bar overhead extension and EZ bar reverse grip curl (3 sets, 10 reps)

Exercise 10: Medicine ball Russian twists (4 sets, 12 reps)

Volume: 32 sets

Thursday: lower body

Exercise 1: Dumbbell goblet squat (5 sets, 5 reps)

Exercise 2: Dumbbell alternating curtsy lunge (4 sets, 6 reps)

Exercise 3: Dumbbell lying leg curl (4 sets, 8 reps)

Exercise 4: Hack squat machine (3 sets, 10 reps)

Exercise 5: Smith machine hip thrust (3 sets, 12 reps)

Exercise 6: Smith machine lunge pulse (3 sets, 15 reps)

Exercise 7: Smith machine calf raise (4 sets, 15 reps)

Volume: 26 sets

Friday: upper body

Exercise 1: Barbell bent-over overhand row (4 sets, 6 reps)

Exercise 2: Dumbbell seated Arnold press (3 sets, 8 reps)

Exercise 3: Barbell decline bench press (3 sets, 8 reps)

Exercise 4: Dumbbell shrug (3 sets, 8 reps)

Exercise 5: Compound set: cable rope straight-arm pulldown and cable rope face pull (3 sets, 10 reps)

Exercise 6: Compound set: cable one-arm side raise and cable one-arm front raise (3 sets, 10 reps)

Exercise 7: Tricep dips (3 sets, 8 reps)

Exercise 8: Dumbbell seated wide curl (3 sets, 8 reps)

Exercise 9: Superset: cable rope overhead extension and cable rope hammer curl (3 sets, 10 reps)

Exercise 10: Hanging leg raise (4 sets, 12 reps)

Volume: 32 sets

Saturday: lower body

Exercise 1: Leg press (5 sets, 5 reps)

Exercise 2: Leg press calf extensions (4 sets, 30 reps)

Exercise 3: Dumbbell Bulgarian split squat (4 sets, 6 reps)

Exercise 4: Barbell Romanian dead lift (4 sets, 8 reps)

Exercise 5: Cable pull-through (3 sets, 10 reps)

Exercise 6: Lying leg curl machine (3 sets, 12 reps)

Exercise 7: Hip abduction machine (3 sets, 15 reps)

Volume: 26 sets

Full Body (Four Days a Week)

Monday

Exercise 1: Barbell back squat (5 sets, 5 reps)

Exercise 2: Dumbbell one-arm row (4 sets, 6 reps)

Exercise 3: Dumbbell seated Arnold press (4 sets, 8 reps)

Exercise 4: Compound set: dumbbell straight-legged dead lift and dumbbell alternating reverse lunge (3 sets, 8 reps)

Exercise 5: Superset: dumbbell close grip bench press and dumbbell chest fly (3 sets, 10 reps)

Exercise 6: Barbell curl (4 sets, 8 reps)

Exercise 7: Reverse machine fly (4 sets, 10 reps)

Exercise 8: Calf raise machine (4 sets, 12 reps)

Exercise 9: Obliques torso twist machine (4 sets, 12 reps)

Volume: 35 sets

Wednesday

Exercise 1: Barbell bench press (5 sets, 5 reps)

Exercise 2: Leg press (4 sets, 6 reps)

Exercise 3: Cable close grip seated low row (4 sets, 8 reps)

Exercise 4: Compound set: dumbbell incline bench press and plate Svend press (3 sets, 8 reps)

Exercise 5: Superset: cable bar front raise and cable bar curl (3 sets, 10 reps)

Exercise 6: Cable bar close grip upright row (4 sets, 8 reps)

Exercise 7: Cable rope glute pull-through (4 sets, 10 reps)

Exercise 8: Cable rope pushdown (4 sets, 12 reps)

Exercise 9: Kneeling cable crunch (4 sets, 12 reps)

Volume: 35 sets

Friday

Exercise 1: Barbell dead lift (5 sets, 5 reps)

Exercise 2: Barbell decline bench press (4 sets, 6 reps)

Exercise 3: Dumbbell seated shoulder press (4 sets, 8 reps)

Exercise 4: Compound set: wide-grip lat pulldown and straight-arm pull-down (3 sets, 8 reps)

Exercise 5: Superset: dumbbell goblet squat and dumbbell overhead extension (3 sets, 10 reps)

Exercise 6: Seated dumbbell alternating hammer curl (4 sets, 8 reps)

Exercise 7: Dumbbell reverse fly (4 sets, 10 reps)

Exercise 8: Lying leg curl machine (4 sets, 12 reps)

Exercise 9: Hanging leg raises (4 sets, 12 reps)

Volume: 35 sets

Sunday

Exercise 1: Barbell overhead press (5 sets, 5 reps)

Exercise 2: Barbell alternating forward lunge (4 sets, 6 reps)

Exercise 3: Barbell bent-over overhand row (4 sets, 8 reps)

Exercise 4: Compound set: dumbbell side raise and dumbbell front raise (3 sets, 8 reps)

Exercise 5: Superset: dumbbell bench press and dumbbell skull crusher (3 sets, 10 reps)

Exercise 6: Dumbbell seated wide curl (4 sets, 8 reps)

Exercise 7: Dumbbell shrugs (4 sets, 10 reps)

Exercise 8: Calf extension machine (4 sets, 12 reps)

Exercise 9: Medicine ball Russian twists (4 sets, 12 reps)

Volume: 35 sets

You can find additional resources at
https://www.emilyrudow.com/findyourstride/resources.

Notes

Introduction

1. Nat Eliason, "Decomplication: How to Find Simple Solutions to 'Hard' Problems," *Nat Eliason* (blog), August 2, 2016, https://www.nateliason.com/blog/decomplication.
2. 50 Cent and Robert Greene, *The 50th Law* (London: HarperCollins, 2009), 66.

Chapter 1

1. Carol Dweck, *Mindset: The New Psychology of Success* (New York: Ballantine Books, 2006).
2. Dweck, *Mindset*, 6.
3. I would be remiss to forego mentioning that some people are more genetically gifted than others when it comes to our metabolisms, ability to put on muscle/size, gaining or losing weight, and so on. However, my point is that we shouldn't use this belief as an excuse for not taking action and accountability for our own fitness efforts.
4. Dweck, *Mindset*, 7.
5. Adam Grant, *Think Again: The Power of Knowing What You Don't Know* (New York: Penguin Random House, 2021), 2.
6. Steve Pavlina, "Driven by Curiosity," *Steve Pavlina* (blog), January 27, 2021, https://stevepavlina.com/blog/2021/01/driven-by-curiosity.
7. Ryan Holiday, *Ego Is the Enemy* (New York: Penguin Random House, 2016), 8.
8. Ryan Holiday, "The Experimental Life: An Introduction to Michel de Montaigne," *Tim Ferriss Show*, October 19, 2010, https://tim.blog/2010/10/19/michel-de-montaigne.

Chapter 2

1. This is a workout video from the 1980s. If you haven't seen it already, I encourage you to check it out, at https://www.youtube.com/watch?v=sWjTnBmCHTY. Just a heads-up: It *burns*.

2. Edward L. Deci and Richard M. Ryan, "The 'What' and 'Why' of Goal Pursuits: Human Needs and the Self-Determination of Behavior," *Psychological Inquiry* 11, no. 4 (2000): 227–268.

3. E. L. Deci and R. M. Ryan, "Commentaries on the 'What' and 'Why' of Goal Pursuits: Human Needs and the Self-Determination of Behavior," *Psychological Inquiry* 11, no. 4 (2000): 269–318.

4. Michelle L. Segar, *No Sweat: How the Simple Science of Motivation Can Bring You a Lifetime of Fitness* (New York: AMACOM, 2015), 37–38.

5. Segar, *No Sweat*, 19.

Chapter 3

1. James Clear, "How to Start New Habits That Actually Stick," *James Clear* (blog), accessed December 14, 2021, https://jamesclear.com/three-steps-habit-change.

2. Steven Pressfield, *The War of Art: Break Through the Blocks and Win Your Inner Creative Battles* (New York: Rugged Land, 2002), 5.

3. Twyla Tharp, *The Creative Habit* (New York: Simon and Schuster, 2003), 14.

4. L. Alison Phillips, Pier-Éric Chamberland, Eric B. Hekler, Jessica Abrams, and Miriam H. Eisenberg, "Intrinsic Rewards Predict Exercise via Behavioral Intentions for Initiators but via Habit Strength for Maintainers," *Sport, Exercise, and Performance Psychology* 5, no. 4 (2016): 352–364.

5. We get more into supplements later in the book, but I wanted to call out that BCAAs are not a necessary supplement (most fitness experts say they're a waste of money). I personally love the added caffeine and deliciousness of BCAAs, so I buy them.

6. K. Milkman, J. Minson, and K. Volpp, "Holding the Hunger Games Hostage at the Gym: An Evaluation of Temptation Bundling," Wharton School Research Paper no. 45, June 6, 2013, https://papers.ssrn.com/sol3/papers.cfm?abstract_id=2183859.

7. P. Lally, C. H. Van Jaarsveld, H. W. Potts, and J. Wardle, "How Are Habits Formed: Modelling Habit Formation in the Real World," *European Journal of Social Psychology* 40, no. 6 (2009): 998–1009.

8. I've created a protein reference guide for you that's available on my website, at https://www.emilyrudow.com/findyourstride/resources.

Chapter 4

1. "It's January 7: Are You Sticking to Your New Year's Resolution?" Wharton School, January 7, 2013, https://knowledge.wharton.upenn.edu/article/its-january-7-are-you-sticking-to-your-new-years-resolution/.

2. Chris Bailey, "Setting Goals Is Largely Overrated," *A Life of Productivity*, January 21, 2021, https://alifeofproductivity.com/setting-goals-is-largely-overrated/.

3. James Clear, "Forget about Setting Goals: Focus on This Instead," *James Clear*, accessed September 27, 2021, https://jamesclear.com/goals-systems.

4. Brad Stulberg, "The Benefits of Focusing on Principles Instead of Goals," *Growth Equation*, accessed September 27, 2021, https://thegrowtheq.com/the-benefits-of-focusing-on-principles-instead-of-goals/.

5. Be careful with numerical KPIs. I discuss my preferred and recommended method for tracking fitness progress in Part III.

6. Nassim Nicholas Taleb, *Antifragile: Things That Gain from Disorder* (New York: Random House, 2014), 303.

7. Taleb, *Antifragile*, 305.

8. Brad Stulberg, "Don't Worry about Being the Best: Worry about Being the Best at Getting Better," *Medium*, September 3, 2017, https://medium.com/personal-growth/dont-worry-about-being-the-best-worry-about-being-the-best-at-getting-better-2ea56b89577e.

Chapter 5

1. James A. Levine, Mark W. Vander Weg, James O. Hill, and Robert C. Klesges, "Non-exercise Activity Thermogenesis: The Crouching Tiger Hidden Dragon of Societal Weight Gain," *Arteriosclerosis, Thrombosis, and Vascular Biology* 26, no. 4 (2006): 729–736.

2. Joe Schwarcz, "How Is the Caloric Value of Food Determined?" McGill University Office for Science and Society, September 6, 2018, https://www.mcgill.ca/oss/article/nutrition/how-caloric-value-food-determined.

3. James L. Hargrove, "History of the Calorie in Nutrition," *Journal of Nutrition* 136, no. 12 (2006), https://doi.org/10.1093/jn/136.12.2957.

4. Hargrove, "History of the Calorie in Nutrition."

5. Schwarcz, "How Is the Caloric Value of Food Determined?"

6. Hargrove, "History of the Calorie in Nutrition."

7. David Benton and Hayley A. Young, "Reducing Calorie Intake May Not Help You Lose Body Weight," *Perspectives on Psychological Science* 12, no. 5 (2017), https://doi:10.1177/1745691617690878.

8. Sabrina Strings, *Fearing the Black Body: The Racial Origins of Fat Phobia* (New York: New York University Press, 2019), 202.

9. Strings, *Fearing the Black Body*, 202.

10. Harvard T. H. Chan School of Public Health, "Ethnic Differences in BMI and Disease Risk," *Obesity Prevention Source*, accessed December 17, 2021, https://www.hsph.harvard.edu/obesity-prevention-source/ethnic-differences-in-bmi-and-disease-risk.

11. Peter T. Katzmarzyk, George A. Bray, Frank L. Greenway, William D. Johnson, Robert L. Newton Jr., Eric Ravussin, Donna H. Ryan, and Claude Bouchard, "Ethnic-Specific BMI and Waist Circumference Thresholds," *Obesity* 19, no. 6 (2011): 1272–1278.

12. Dennis Thompson, "Study: Black Women Lose Less Weight Than White Women on Same Diet," *MedicineNet*, December 19, 2013, https://www.medicinenet.com/script/main/art.asp?articlekey=175844; Shereen Jegtvig, "African American Women Have a Harder Time Losing Weight," *Reuters*, January 3, 2014, https://www.reuters.com/article/us-african-american-women-weight-idUSBREA020TH20140103.

13. Carly Stern, "Why BMI Is a Flawed Health Standard, Especially for People of Color," *Washington Post*, May 5, 2021, https://www.washingtonpost.com/lifestyle/wellness/healthy-bmi-obesity-race-/2021/05/04/655390f0-ad0d-11eb-acd3-24b44a57093a_story.html.

14. Christopher Barakat, Jeremy Pearson, Guillermo Escalante, Bill Campbell, and Eduardo O. De Souza, "Body Recomposition: Can Trained Individuals Build Muscle and Lose Fat at the Same Time?" *Strength and Conditioning Journal* 42, no. 5 (2020): 7–21.

15. Antonio Paoli, Keith Grimaldi, Dominic D'Agostino, Lorenzo Cenci, Tatiana Moro, Antonino Bianco, and Antonio Palma, "Ketogenic Diet Does Not Affect Strength Performance in Elite Artistic Gymnasts," *Journal of the International Society of Sports Nutrition* 9, no. 1 (2012), https://doi:10.1186/1550-2783-9-34.

16. Ina Garthe, Truls Raastad, Per Egil Refsnes, Anu Koivisto, and Jorunn Sundgot-Borgen, "Effect of Two Different Weight-Loss Rates on Body Composition and Strength and Power-Related Performance in Elite Athletes," *International Journal of Sport Nutrition and Exercise Metabolism* 21, no. 2 (2011): 97–104.

17. Menno Henselmans, "Can You Gain Muscle and Lose Fat at the Same Time?" *Menno Henselmans* (blog), accessed October 20, 2021, https://mennohenselmans.com/gain-muscle-and-lose-fat-at-the-same-time/.

Chapter 6

1. James A. Levine, Mark W. Vander Weg, James O. Hill, and Robert C. Klesges, "Non-exercise Activity Thermogenesis: The Crouching Tiger Hidden Dragon of Societal Weight Gain," *Arteriosclerosis, Thrombosis, and Vascular Biology* 26, no. 4 (2006): 729–736.

2. Paul Revlia, "How to Calculate Maintenance Calories: 2 Ways," *YouTube*, January 30, 2020, https://www.youtube.com/watch?v=J5YKmWf3a90.

3. Personal Trainer Collective, "How to Work Out Maintenance Calories with Eric Helms: Do BMR Calculators Work?" *YouTube*, January 22, 2018, https://www.youtube.com/watch?v=4h9dhQUZECk.

4. M. D. Mifflin, S. T. St. Jeor, L. A. Hill, B. J. Scott, S. A. Daugherty, and Y. O. Koh, "A New Predictive Equation for Resting Energy Expenditure in Healthy Individuals," *American Journal of Clinical Nutrition* 51, no. 2 (1990): 241–247.

5. Anna Shcherbina, C. M. Mattsson, Daryl Waggott, Heidi Salisbury, Jeffrey W. Christle, Trevor Hastie, Matthew T. Wheeler, and Euan A. Ashley, "Accuracy in Wrist-Worn, Sensor-Based Measurements of Heart Rate and Energy Expenditure in a Diverse Cohort," *Journal of Personalized Medicine* 7, no. 2 (2017): 3.

Chapter 7

1. John Romaniello, "Why You Need to Stop Overthinking Your Training," *Roman Fitness Systems*, accessed November 16, 2021, https://romanfitnesssystems.com/articles/why-you-need-to-stop-overthinking-your-training/.

2. P. Li, Y. L. Yin, D. Li, S. W. Kim, and G. Wu, "Amino Acids and Immune Function," *British Journal of Nutrition* 98, no. 2 (2007): 237–252.

3. L. Lee Hamm, Nazih Nakhoul, and Kathleen S. Hering-Smith, "Acid-Base Homeostasis," *Clinical Journal of the American Society of Nephrology* 10, no. 12 (2015): 2232–2242.

4. Ayako Hashimoto and Taiho Kambe, "Mg, Zn and Cu Transport Proteins: A Brief Overview from Physiological and Molecular Perspectives," suppl., *Journal of Nutritional Science and Vitaminology* (Tokyo) 61 (2015): S116–S118.

5. Dominik H. Pesta and Varman T. Samuel, "A High-Protein Diet for Reducing Body Fat: Mechanisms and Possible Caveats," *Nutrition and Metabolism* 11, no. 1 (2014): 53.

6. A. M. Johnstone, R. J. Stubbs, and C. G. Harbron, "Effect of Overfeeding Macronutrients on Day-to-Day Food Intake in Man," *European Journal of Clinical Nutrition* 50, no. 7 (1996): 418–430.

7. Thomas L. Halton and Frank B. Hu, "The Effects of High Protein Diets on Thermogenesis, Satiety and Weight Loss: A Critical Review," *Journal of the American College of Nutrition* 23, no. 5 (2004): 373–385.

8. Douglas Paddon-Jones, Eric Westman, Richard D. Mattes, Robert R. Wolfe, Arne Astrup, and Margriet Westerterp-Plantenga, "Protein, Weight Management, and Satiety," *American Journal of Clinical Nutrition* 87, no. 5 (2008): 1558S–1561S.

9. Robert W. Morton, Kevin T. Murphy, Sean R. McKellar, Brad J. Schoenfeld, Menno Henselmans, Eric Helms, Alan A. Aragon, et al., "A Systematic Review, Meta-analysis and Meta-Regression of the Effect of Protein Supplementation on Resistance Training-Induced Gains in Muscle Mass and Strength in Healthy Adults," *British Journal of Sports Medicine* 52, no. 6 (2018): 376–384.

10. Jeff Nippard, "The Science behind My High Protein Diet (How Much Per Day for Muscle Growth and Fat Loss?)," *YouTube*, November 16, 2019, https://www.youtube.com/watch?v=g82MXEJC3NI.

11. Amy J. Hector and Stuart M. Phillips, "Protein Recommendations for Weight Loss in Elite Athletes: A Focus on Body Composition and Performance," *International Journal of Sport Nutrition and Exercise Metabolism* 28, no. 2 (2018), https://pubmed.ncbi.nlm.nih.gov/29182451.

12. Hector and Phillips, "Protein Recommendations."

13. Menno Henselmans, "Eric Helms and Protein: A Research Review," *Menno Henselmans* (blog), accessed November 12, 2021, https://mennohenselmans.com/eric-helms-protein.

14. "Too Much Protein May Cause Reduced Kidney Function," *Harvard Gazette*, March 13, 2003, https://news.harvard.edu/gazette/story/2003/03/too-much-protein-may-cause-reduced-kidney-function/.

15. Michaela C. Devries, Arjun Sithamparapillai, K. Scott Brimble, Laura Banfield, Robert W. Morton, and Stuart M. Phillips, "Changes in Kidney Function Do Not Differ between Healthy Adults Consuming Higher- Compared with Lower- or Normal-Protein Diets: A Systematic Review and Meta-analysis," *Journal of Nutrition* 148 no. 11 (2018): 1760–1775.

16. Jay J. Cao, "High Dietary Protein Intake and Protein-Related Acid Load on Bone Health," *Current Osteoporosis Reports* 15 no. 6 (2017): 571–576.

17. Marissa M. Shams-White, Mei Chung, Mengxi Du, Zhuxuan Fu, Karl L. Insogna, Micaela C. Karlsen, Meryl S. LeBoff, et al., "Dietary Protein and Bone Health: A Systematic Review and Meta-analysis from the National Osteoporosis Foundation," *American Journal of Clinical Nutrition* 105, no. 6 (2017), https://doi.org/10.3945/ajcn.116.145110.

18. Jose Antonio, Anya Ellerbroek, Tobin Silver, Steve Orris, Max Scheiner, Adriana Gonzalez, and Corey A. Peacock, "A High Protein Diet (3.4 g/kg/d) Combined with a Heavy Resistance Training Program Improves Body Composition in Healthy Trained Men and Women—a Follow-Up Investigation," *Journal of the International Society of Sports Nutrition* 12, no. 39 (2015), https://doi.org/10.1186/s12970-015-0100-0.

19. David S. Ludwig, Frank B. Hu, Luc Tappy, and Jennie Brand-Miller, "Dietary Carbohydrates: Role of Quality and Quantity in Chronic Disease," *BMJ* 361 (June 2018), https://www.bmj.com/content/361/bmj.k2340.

20. "Monosaccharide," *Encyclopedia Britannica*, accessed October 11, 2021, https://www.britannica.com/science/monosaccharide.

21. "Oligosaccharide," *Encyclopedia Britannica*, accessed October 11, 2021, https://www.britannica.com/science/oligosaccharide.

22. Julie E. Holesh, Sanah Aslam, and Andrew Martin, "Physiology, Carbohydrates," *StatPearls*, July 26, 2021, https://www.ncbi.nlm.nih.gov/books/NBK459280/.

23. Philipp Mergenthaler, Ute Lindauer, Gerald A. Dienel, and Andreas Meisel, "Sugar for the Brain: The Role of Glucose in Physiological and Pathological Brain Function," *Trends in Neurosciences* 36, no. 10 (2013): 587–597.

24. James M. Lattimer and Mark D Haub, "Effects of Dietary Fiber and Its Components on Metabolic Health," *Nutrients* 2, no. 12 (2010): 1266–1289.

25. Lattimer and Haub, "Effects of Dietary Fiber."

26. B. J. Venn and T. J. Green, "Glycemic Index and Glycemic Load: Measurement Issues and Their Effect on Diet-Disease Relationships," suppl. 1, *European Journal of Clinical Nutrition* 61 (2007): S122–S131.

27. Menno Henselmans, "The Science of Nutrition: Is a Carb a Carb?" *Simply Shredded*, accessed November 12, 2021, https://simplyshredded.com/the-science-of-nutrition-is-a-carb-a-carb.html.

28. "Dieting: The Drinking Man's Danger," *Time,* March 5, 1965, http://content.time.com/time/subscriber/article/0,33009,839328-1,00.html.

29. Ghanim Salih Mahdi, "The Atkin's Diet Controversy," *Annals of Saudi Medicine* 26, no. 3 (2006): 244–245.

30. David S. Ludwig and Cara B. Ebbeling, "The Carbohydrate-Insulin Model of Obesity: Beyond 'Calories In, Calories Out,'" *JAMA Internal Medicine* 178, no. 8 (2018), https://www.ncbi.nlm.nih.gov/pmc/articles/PMC6082688.

31. Sander Kersten, "Mechanisms of Nutritional and Hormonal Regulation of Lipogenesis," *EMBO Reports* 2, no. 4 (2001): 282–286.

32. Kevin D. Hall and Juen Guo, "Obesity Energetics: Body Weight Regulation and the Effects of Diet Composition," *Gastroenterology* 152, no. 7 (2017), https://www.ncbi.nlm.nih.gov/pmc/articles/PMC5568065.

33. Andrea C. Buchholz and Dale A. Schoeller, "Is a Calorie a Calorie?" *American Journal of Clinical Nutrition* 79, no. 5 (2004): 899S–906S.

34. Ludwig et al., "Dietary Carbohydrates."

35. Menno Henselmans, "Do Strength Trainees Really Need Carbs?" *Menno Henselmans* (blog), accessed November 12, 2021, https://mennohenselmans.com/do-strength-trainees-really-need-carbs.

36. Jennifer Wismann and Darryn Willoughby, "Gender Differences in Carbohydrate Metabolism and Carbohydrate Loading," *Journal of the International Society of Sports Nutrition* 3, no. 1 (2006): 28–34.

37. Mark A. Tarnopolsky, "Sex Differences in Exercise Metabolism and the Role of 17-Beta Estradiol," *Medicine and Science in Sports and Exercise* 40, no. 4 (2008): 648–654.

38. Mark A. Tarnopolsky, Carol Zawada, Lindsay B. Richmond, Sherry Carter, Jane Shearer, Terry Graham, and Stuart M. Phillips, "Gender Differences in Carbohydrate Loading Are Related to Energy Intake," *Journal of Applied Physiology* 91, no. 1 (2001): 225–230.

39. Gloria Hernández Alcantara, Arturo Jiménez Cruz, Montserrat Bacardí Gascón, "Effect of Low Carbohydrate Diets on Weight Loss and Glycosilated Hemoglobin in People with Type 2 Diabetes: Systematic Review," *Nutricion Hospitalaria* 32, no. 5 (2015): 1960–1966.

40. John Fawkes, "How to Eat According to Your Carb Tolerance," *Better Humans*, December 28, 2018, https://betterhumans.pub/how-to-eat-according-to-your-carb-tolerance-eac3c70f2f3d.

41. Fawkes, "How to Eat."

42. Mads F. Hjorth, Christian Ritz, Ellen E. Blaak, Wim H. M. Saris, Dominique Langin, Sanne Kellebjerg Poulsen, Thomas Meinert Larsen, Thorkild I. A. Sorensen, Yishai Zohar, and Arne Astrup, "Pretreatment Fasting Plasma Glucose and Insulin Modify Dietary Weight Loss Success: Results from 3 Randomized Clinical Trials," *American Journal of Clinical Nutrition* 106, no. 2 (2017): 499–505.

43. Walter C. Willett and Rudolph L. Leibel, "Dietary Fat Is Not a Major Determinant of Body Fat," suppl. 9B, *American Journal of Medicine* 113 (2002): 47S–59S.

44. Ann F. La Berge, "How the Ideology of Low Fat Conquered America," *Journal of the History of Medicine and Allied Sciences* 63, no. 2 (April 2008): 139–177.

45. Patty W. Siri-Tarino, Qi Sun, Frank B. Hu, and Ronald M. Krauss, "Meta-analysis of Prospective Cohort Studies Evaluating the Association of Saturated Fat with Cardiovascular Disease," *American Journal of Clinical Nutrition* 91, no. 3 (2010): 535–546.

46. PREDIMED, "Dietary Fat Intake and Risk of Cardiovascular Disease and All-Cause Mortality in a Population at High Risk of Cardiovascular Disease," *American Journal of Clinical Nutrition* 102, no. 6 (December 2015): 1563–1573.

47. Tracey Phillips, April C. Childs, Darlene M. Dreon, Stephen Phinney, and Christiaan Leeuwenburgh, "A Dietary Supplement Attenuates IL-6 and CRP after Eccentric Exercise in Untrained Males," *Medicine and Science in Sports and Exercise* 35, no. 12 (2003): 2032–2037.

48. Harvard Health Publishing, "The Truth about Fats: The Good, the Bad, and the In-Between," December 11, 2019, https://www.health.harvard.edu/staying-healthy/the-truth-about-fats-bad-and-good.

49. Peter J. Abernethy, Robert Thayer, and Albert W. Taylor, "Acute and Chronic Responses of Skeletal Muscle to Endurance and Sprint Exercise: A Review," *Sports Medicine* 10, no. 6 (1990), https://link.springer.com/article/10.2165/00007256-199010060-00004.

50. Lonnie M. Lowery, "Dietary Fat and Sports Nutrition: A Primer," *Journal of Sports Science and Medicine* 3, no. 3 (2004), https://www.ncbi.nlm.nih.gov/pmc/articles/PMC3905293/.

51. A. Schek, H. Braun, A. Carlsohn, M. Großhauser, D. König, A. Lampen, S. Mosler, et al., "Position of the Working Group Sports Nutrition of the German Nutrition Society (DGE): Fats, Fat Loading, and Sports Performance," *German Journal of Sports Medicine* 71 (2020): 199–207.

52. Eric C. Westman, William S. Yancy Jr., John C. Mavropoulos, Megan Marquart, and Jennifer R. McDuffie, "The Effect of a Low-Carbohydrate, Ketogenic Diet versus a Low-Glycemic Index Diet on Glycemic Control in Type 2 Diabetes Mellitus," *Nutrition and Metabolism* 5 (2008), https://pubmed.ncbi.nlm.nih.gov/19099589/.

53. Kristin W. Barañano and Adam L Hartman, "The Ketogenic Diet: Uses in Epilepsy and Other Neurologic Illnesses," *Current Treatment Options in Neurology* 10, no. 6 (2008): 410–419.

54. Caryn Zinn, Matthew Wood, Mikki Williden, Simon Chatterton, and Ed Maunder, "Ketogenic Diet Benefits Body Composition and Well-Being but Not Performance in a Pilot Case Study of New Zealand Endurance Athletes," *Journal of the International Society of Sports Nutrition* 14, no. 22 (2017), https://doi.org/10.1186/s12970-017-0180-0.

55. Ann G. Liu, Nikki A. Ford, Frank B. Hu, Kathleen M. Zelman, Dariush Mozaffarian, and Penny M. Kris-Etherton, "A Healthy Approach to Dietary Fats: Understanding the Science and Taking Action to Reduce Consumer Confusion," *Nutrition Journal* 16, no. 1 (2017), https://www.ncbi.nlm.nih.gov/pmc/articles/PMC5577766/.

56. "Scurvy Is Still a Thing in Canada," McMaster University, January 20, 2020, https://healthsci.mcmaster.ca/home/2020/01/20/scurvy-is-still-a-thing-in-canada.

57. World Health Organization and Centers for Disease Control and Prevention, *Assessing the Iron Status of Populations*, 2nd ed. (Geneva, Switzerland: World Health Organization, 2007).

58. Saeed Akhtar, Anwaar Ahmed, Muhammad Atif Randhawa, Sunethra Atukorala, Nimmathota Arlappa, Tariq Ismail, and Zulfiqar Ali, "Prevalence of Vitamin A Deficiency in South Asia: Causes, Outcomes, and Possible Remedies," *Journal of Health, Population, and Nutrition* 31, no. 4 (2013), https://pubmed.ncbi.nlm.nih.gov/24592582/.

59. Gerry K. Schwalfenberg and Stephen J. Genuis, "The Importance of Magnesium in Clinical Healthcare," *Scientifica* (Cairo) 2017 (2017), https://pubmed.ncbi.nlm.nih.gov/29093983.

60. Rebecca B. Costello, Ronald J. Elin, Andrea Rosanoff, Taylor C. Wallace, Fernando Guerrero-Romero, Adela Hruby, Pamela L. Lutsey, et al., "Perspective: The Case for an Evidence-Based Reference Interval for Serum Magnesium: The Time Has Come," *Advances in Nutrition* 7, no. 6 (2016): 977–993.

61. James J. DiNicolantonio, James H. O'Keefe, and William Wilson, "Subclinical Magnesium Deficiency: A Principal Driver of Cardiovascular Disease and a Public Health Crisis," *Open Heart* 5, no. 1 (2018), https://pubmed.ncbi.nlm.nih.gov/29387426/.

62. E. Gür, O. Ercan, G. Can, S. Akkuş, S. Güzelöz, S. Ciftcili, A. Arvas, and O. Iltera, "Prevalence and Risk Factors of Iodine Deficiency among Schoolchildren," *Journal of Tropical Pediatrics* 49, no. 3 (2003): 168–171.

63. Vaughan Somerville, Cameron Bringans, and Andrea Braakhuis, "Polyphenols and Performance: A Systematic Review and Meta-analysis," *Sports Medicine* 47 (2017): 1589–1599.

64. Jason E. Tang, Daniel R. Moore, Gregory W. Kujbida, Mark A. Tarnopolsky, and Stuart M. Phillips, "Ingestion of Whey Hydrolysate, Casein, or Soy Protein Isolate: Effects on Mixed Muscle Protein Synthesis at Rest and Following Resistance Exercise in Young Men," *Journal of Applied Physiology* 107, no. 3 (2009): 987–992.

65. Nicolas Babault, Christos Païzis, Gaëlle Deley, Laetitia Guérin-Deremaux, Marie-Hélène Saniez, Catherine Lefranc-Millot, and François A. Allaert, "Pea Proteins Oral Supplementation Promotes Muscle Thickness Gains during Resistance Training: A Double-Blind, Randomized, Placebo-Controlled Clinical Trial vs. Whey Protein," *Journal of the International Society of Sports Nutrition* 12, no. 1 (2015), https://jissn.biomedcentral.com/articles/10.1186/s12970-014-0064-5.

66. Jose Antonio and Victoria Ciccone, "The Effects of Pre versus Post Workout Supplementation of Creatine Monohydrate on Body Composition and Strength," *Journal of the International Society of Sports Nutrition* 10 (2013), https://pubmed.ncbi.nlm.nih.gov/23919405/.

67. S. Ryu, S. K. Choi, S. S. Joung, H. Suh, Y. S. Cha, S. Lee, and K. Lim, "Caffeine as a Lipolytic Food Component Increases Endurance Performance in Rats and Athletes," *Journal of Nutritional Science and Vitaminology* (Tokyo) 47, no. 2 (2001): 139–146.

68. K. Collomp, S. Ahmaidi, J. C. Chatard, M. Audran, and C. Préfaut, "Benefits of Caffeine Ingestion on Sprint Performance in Trained and Untrained Swimmers," *European Journal of Applied Physiology and Occupational Physiology* 64, no. 4 (1992), https://pubmed.ncbi.nlm.nih.gov/1592065.

69. Matthew S. Ganio, Jennifer F. Klau, Douglas J. Casa, Lawrence E. Armstrong, and Carl M. Maresh, "Effect of Caffeine on Sport-Specific Endurance Performance: A Systematic Review," *Journal of Strength and Conditioning Research* 23, no. 1 (2009): 315–324.

70. J. D. Wiles, S. R. Bird, J. Hopkins, and M. Riley, "Effect of Caffeinated Coffee on Running Speed, Respiratory Factors, Blood Lactate and Perceived Exertion During 1500-M Treadmill Running," *British Journal of Sports Medicine* 26, no. 2 (1992): 116–120.

71. Gordon L. Warren, Nicole D. Park, Robert D. Maresca, Kimberly I. McKibans, and Melinda L. Millard-Stafford, "Effect of Caffeine Ingestion on Muscular Strength and Endurance: A Meta-analysis," *Medicine and Science in Sports and Exercise* 42, no. 7 (2010): 1375–1387.

72. US Food and Drug Administration, "Pure and Highly Concentrated Caffeine," March 30, 2021, https://www.fda.gov/food/dietary-supplement-products-ingredients/pure-and-highly-concentrated-caffeine.

73. Seema B. Jabbar and Mark G. Hanly, "Fatal Caffeine Overdose: A Case Report and Review of Literature," *American Journal of Forensic Medicine and Pathology* 34, no. 4 (2013): 321–324.

74. Erica R. Goldstein, Tim Ziegenfuss, Doug Kalman, Richard Kreider, Bill Campbell, Colin Wilborn, Lem Taylor, et al., "International Society of Sports Nutrition Position Stand: Caffeine and Performance," *Journal of the International Society of Sports Nutrition* 7, no. 1 (2010), https://jissn.biomedcentral.com/articles/10.1186/1550-2783-7-5.

Chapter 8

1. Scott Q. Siler, Richard A. Neese, and Marc K. Hellerstein, "De Novo Lipogenesis, Lipid Kinetics, and Whole-Body Lipid Balances in Humans after Acute Alcohol Consumption," *American Journal of Clinical Nutrition* 70, no. 5 (November 1999): 928–936.

2. Martin R. Yeomans, "Short Term Effects of Alcohol on Appetite in Humans: Effects of Context and Restrained Eating," *Appetite* 55, no. 3 (2010): 565–573.

3. Evelyn B. Parr, Donny M. Camera, Jose L. Areta, Louise M. Burke, Stuart M. Phillips, John A. Hawley, and Vernon G. Coffey, "Alcohol Ingestion Impairs Maximal Post-exercise Rates of Myofibrillar Protein Synthesis Following a Single Bout of Concurrent Training," *PLoS One* 9, no. 2 (2014), https://pubmed.ncbi.nlm.nih.gov/24533082.

4. J. Frias, J. M. Torres, M. T. Miranda, E. Ruiz, and E. Ortega, "Effects of Acute Alcohol Intoxication on Pituitary-Gonadal Axis Hormones, Pituitary-Adrenal Axis Hormones, Beta-Endorphin and Prolactin in Human Adults of Both Sexes," *Alcohol and Alcoholism* (Oxford) 37, no. 2 (March–April 2002): 169–173.

Chapter 9

1. G. B. Forbes, "Body Fat Content Influences the Body Composition Response to Nutrition and Exercise," *Annals of the New York Academy of Sciences* 904 (May 2000): 359–365.

2. Eric Trexler, "Should You Cut Before You Bulk? How Body-Fat Levels Affect Your P-Ratio," *Stronger by Science*, February 8, 2021, https://www.strongerbyscience.com/p-ratios/.

3. Eric R. Helms, Alan A. Aragon, and Peter J. Fitschen, "Evidence-Based Recommendations for Natural Bodybuilding Contest Preparation: Nutrition and Supplementation," *Journal of the International Society of Sports Nutrition* 11, no. 20 (2014), https://doi.org/10.1186/1550-2783-11-20.

4. Asli Devrim, Pelin Bilgic, and Nobuko Hongu, "Is There Any Relationship between Body Image Perception, Eating Disorders, and Muscle Dysmorphic Disorders in Male Bodybuilders?" *American Journal of Men's Health* 12, no. 5 (September 2018): 1746–1758.

5. Mike Thurston, "Nutrition Basics: The Lean Bulk," *YouTube*, January 22, 2017, https://www.youtube.com/watch?v=Ci3qXtNFU_w.

6. Juma Iraki, Peter Fitschen, Sergio Espinar, and Eric Helms, "Nutrition Recommendations for Bodybuilders in the Off-Season: A Narrative Review," *Sports* (Basel, Switzerland) 7, no. 7 (2019), https://www.ncbi.nlm.nih.gov/pmc/articles/PMC6680710.

7. Ina Garthe, Truls Raastad, Per Egil Refsnes, and Jorunn Sundgot-Borgen, "Effect of Nutritional Intervention on Body Composition and Performance in Elite Athletes," *European Journal of Sport Science* 13, no. 3 (2013): 295–303.

8. Helms, Aragon, and Fitschen, "Evidence-Based Recommendations."

9. E. R. Helms, P. J. Fitschen, A. A. Aragon, J. Cronin, and B. J. Schoenfeld, "Recommendations for Natural Bodybuilding Contest Preparation: Resistance and Cardiovascular Training," *Journal of Sports Medicine and Physical Fitness* 55, no. 3 (March 2015): 164–178.

10. Eric T. Trexler, Abbie E. Smith-Ryan, and Layne E. Norton, "Metabolic Adaptation to Weight Loss: Implications for the Athlete," *Journal of the International Society of Sports Nutrition* 11, no. 1 (2014): 7.

11. Trexler, Smith-Ryan, and Norton, "Metabolic Adaptation."

12. Katey Davidson, "Refeed Day: What It Is and How to Do It," *Healthline*, April 1, 2020, https://www.healthline.com/nutrition/refeed-day.

13. Paul Revelia, "Diet Break What I Have Learned," *YouTube*, January 12, 2018, https://www.youtube.com/watch?v=nf6H4_R5Zxs.

14. N. M. Byrne, A. Sainsbury, N. A. King, A. P. Hills, and R. E. Wood, "Intermittent Energy Restriction Improves Weight Loss Efficiency in Obese Men: The MATADOR Study," *International Journal of Obesity* (London) 42, no. 2 (February 2018): 129–138.

15. Jeff Nippard, "Do Diet Breaks Improve Fat Loss and Metabolism? (New Scientific Research)," *YouTube*, December 3, 2017, https://www.youtube.com/watch?v=TaaA2fsuXZU.

16. Stuart B. Murray, Eva Pila, Jonathon M. Mond, Deborah Mitchison, Aaron J. Blashill, Catherine M. Sabiston, and Scott Griffiths, "Cheat Meals: A Benign or Ominous Variant of Binge Eating Behavior?" *Appetite* 130 (November 2018): 274–278.

17. S. N. Kreitzman, A. Y. Coxon, and K. F. Szaz, "Glycogen Storage: Illusions of Easy Weight Loss, Excessive Weight Regain, and Distortions in Estimates of Body Composition," suppl., *American Journal of Clinical Nutrition* 56, no. 1 (July 1992): 292S–293S.

18. Jay, "When Should I Recalculate My Calorie Intake and Adjust My Diet?" *A Workout Routine*, January 29, 2019, https://www.aworkoutroutine.com/when-to-recalculate-calorie-intake-and-adjust-your-diet/.

19. Mike Rosa, email interview by the author, August 18, 2021.

Chapter 10

1. Robert M. Edinburgh, Helen E. Bradley, Nurul-Fadhilah Abdullah, Scott L. Robinson, Oliver J. Chrzanowski-Smith, Jean-Philippe Walhin, Sophie Joanisse, et al., "Lipid Metabolism Links Nutrient-Exercise Timing to Insulin Sensitivity in Men Classified as Overweight or Obese," *Journal of Clinical Endocrinology and Metabolism* 105, no. 3 (March 2020): 660–676.

2. Northumbria University, "Lose Fat Faster before Breakfast," *ScienceDaily*, January 24, 2013, https://www.sciencedaily.com/releases/2013/01/130124091425.htm.

3. Brad Jon Schoenfeld, Alan Albert Aragon, Colin D. Wilborn, James W. Krieger, and Gul T. Sonmez, "Body Composition Changes Associated with Fasted versus Non-fasted Aerobic Exercise," *Journal of the International Society of Sports Nutrition* 11, no. 1 (2014): 54.

4. K. De Bock, W. Derave, B. O. Eijnde, M. K. Hesselink, E. Koninckx, A. J. Rose, P. Schrauwen, A. Bonen, E. A. Richter, and P. Hespel, "Effect of Training in the Fasted State on Metabolic Responses during Exercise with Carbohydrate Intake," *Journal of Applied Physiology* 104, no. 4 (2008): 1045–1055.

5. Chad Kerksick, Travis Harvey, Jeff Stout, Bill Campbell, Colin Wilborn, Richard Kreider, Doug Kalman et al., "International Society of Sports Nutrition Position Stand: Nutrient Timing," *Journal of the International Society of Sports Nutrition* 5 (October 2008): 17.

6. Stephanie Welton, Robert Minty, Teresa O'Driscoll, Hannah Willms, Denise Poirier, Sharen Madden, and Len Kelly, "Intermittent Fasting and Weight Loss: Systematic Review," *Canadian Family Physician* 66, no. 2 (February 2020): 117–125.

7. Adrienne R. Barnosky, Kristin K. Hoddy, Terry G. Unterman, and Krista A. Varady, "Intermittent Fasting vs. Daily Calorie Restriction for Type 2 Diabetes Prevention: A Review of Human Findings," *Translational Research* 164, no. 4 (2014): 302–311.

8. Leonie K. Heilbronn, Anthony E. Civitarese, Iwona Bogacka, Steven R. Smith, Matthew Hulver, and Eric Ravussin, "Glucose Tolerance and Skeletal Muscle Gene Expression in Response to Alternate Day Fasting," *Obesity Research* 13, no. 3 (March 2005): 574–581.

9. Abdallah Kobeissy, Mira S. Zantout, and Sami T. Azar, "Suggested Insulin Regimens for Patients with Type 1 Diabetes Mellitus Who Wish to Fast during the Month of Ramadan," *Clinical Therapeutics* 30, no. 8 (August 2008): 1408–1415.

10. Kevin D. Tipton, D. Lee Hamilton, and Iain J. Gallagher, "Assessing the Role of Muscle Protein Breakdown in Response to Nutrition and Exercise in Humans," suppl., *Sports Medicine* (Auckland) 48, no. 1 (2018): 53–64.

11. Brad Jon Schoenfeld, Alan Albert Aragon, and James W. Krieger, "The Effect of Protein Timing on Muscle Strength and Hypertrophy: A Meta-analysis," *Journal of the International Society of Sports Nutrition* 10, no. 1 (2013): 53.

12. Jay R. Hoffman, Nicholas A. Ratamess, Christopher P. Tranchina, Stefanie L. Rashti, Jie Kang, and Avery D. Faigenbaum, "Effect of Protein-Supplement Timing on Strength, Power, and Body-Composition Changes in Resistance-Trained Men," *International Journal of Sport Nutrition and Exercise Metabolism* 19, no. 2 (April 2009): 172–185.

13. Aaron W. Staples, Nicholas A. Burd, Daniel W. D. West, Katharine D. Currie, Philip J. Atherton, Daniel R. Moore, Michael J. Rennie, Maureen J. Macdonald, Steven K. Baker, and Stuart M. Phillips, "Carbohydrate Does Not Augment Exercise-Induced Protein Accretion versus Protein Alone," *Medicine and Science in Sports and Exercise* 43, no. 7 (July 2011): 1154–1161.

14. Brian Leutholtz and Chad M. Kerksick, "Nutrient Administration and Resistance Training," *Journal of the International Society of Sports Nutrition* 2, no. 1 (2005): 50–67.

15. Daniel R. Moore, Meghann J. Robinson, Jessica L. Fry, Jason E. Tang, Elisa I. Glover, Sarah B. Wilkinson, Todd Prior, Mark A. Tarnopolsky, and Stuart M. Phillips, "Ingested Protein Dose Response of Muscle and Albumin Protein Synthesis after Resistance Exercise in Young Men," *American Journal of Clinical Nutrition* 89, no. 1 (2009): 161–168.

16. William Kyle Mitchell, Beth E. Phillips, John P. Williams, Debbie Rankin, Jonathan N. Lund, Kenneth Smith, and Philip J. Atherton, "A Dose- Rather Than Delivery Profile–Dependent Mechanism Regulates the 'Muscle-Full' Effect in Response to Oral Essential Amino Acid Intake in Young Men," *Journal of Nutrition* 145, no. 2 (February 2015): 207–214.

17. Kerksick et al., "International Society of Sports Nutrition Position Stand."

Chapter 11

1. Chrissy King, "Racism Needs to Be Part of the Conversation about Dismantling Diet Culture," *Shape*, February 9, 2021, https://www.shape.com/lifestyle/mind-and-body/racism-diet-culture.

2. Joachim Westenhoefer, Albert J. Stunkard, and Volker Pudel, "Validation of the Flexible and Rigid Control Dimensions of Dietary Restraint," *International Journal of Eating Disorders* 26, no. 1 (1999): 53–64.

3. Joachim Westenhoefer, B. von Falck, A. Stellfeldt, and S. Fintelmann, "Behavioural Correlates of Successful Weight Reduction over 3 Y. Results from the Lean Habits Study," *International Journal of Obesity and Related Metabolic Disorders* 28, no. 2 (2004): 334–335.

4. Joachim Westenhoefer, Daniel Engel, Claus Holst, Jürgen Lorenz, Matthew Peacock, James Stubbs, Stephen Whybrow, and Monique Raats, "Cognitive and Weight-Related Correlates of Flexible and Rigid Restrained Eating Behavior," *Eating Behaviors* 14, no. 1 (2013): 69–72.

5. C. F. Smith, D. A. Williamson, G. A. Bray, and D. H. Ryan, "Flexible vs. Rigid Dieting Strategies: Relationship with Adverse Behavioral Outcomes," *Appetite* 32, no. 3 (1999): 295–305.

6. Jeff Nippard, "Why You Shouldn't Eat Clean: How to Lose Fat More Effectively," *YouTube*, August 16, 2020, https://www.youtube.com/watch?v=ytN366VCGls.

7. Ahmed Ismaeel, Suzy Weems, and Darryn S. Willoughby, "A Comparison of the Nutrient Intakes of Macronutrient-Based Dieting and Strict Dieting Bodybuilders," *International Journal of Sport Nutrition and Exercise Metabolism* 28, no. 5 (2018): 502–508.

8. Tiffany M. Stewart, Donald A. Williamson, and Marney A. White, "Rigid vs. Flexible Dieting: Association with Eating Disorder Symptoms in Nonobese Women," *Appetite* 38, no. 1 (2002): 39–44.

9. Nancy S. Koven and Alexandra W. Abry, "The Clinical Basis of Orthorexia Nervosa: Emerging Perspectives," *Neuropsychiatric Disease and Treatment* 11 (February 2015): 385–394.

10. Evelyn Tribole and Elyse Resch, *Intuitive Eating: A Revolutionary Program That Works* (New York: St. Martin's Griffin, 2012), 45.

11. Tribole and Resch, *Intuitive Eating*, 46–54.

Chapter 12

1. Jean Harvey, Rebecca Krukowski, Jeff Priest, and Delia West, "Log Often, Lose More: Electronic Dietary Self-Monitoring for Weight Loss," *Obesity* 27 (2019): 380–384.

2. Pauline Ducrot, Caroline Méjean, Vani Aroumougame, Gladys Ibanez, Benjamin Allès, Emmanuelle Kesse-Guyot, Serge Hercberg, and Sandrine Péneau, "Meal Planning Is Associated with Food Variety, Diet Quality and Body Weight Status in a Large Sample of French Adults," *International Journal of Behavioral Nutrition and Physical Activity* 14, no. 1 (2017): 12.

3. Dennis Thompson, "Study: Black Women Lose Less Weight Than White Women on Same Diet," *MedicineNet*, December 19, 2014, https://www.medicinenet.com/script/main/art.asp?articlekey=175844.

4. Christina F. Haughton, Valerie J. Silfee, Monica L. Wang, Andrea C. Lopez-Cepero, David P. Estabrook, Christine Frisard, Milagros C. Rosal, Sherry L. Pagoto, and Stephenie C. Lemon, "Racial/Ethnic Representation in Lifestyle Weight Loss Intervention Studies in the United States: A Systematic Review," *Preventive Medicine Reports* 9 (March 2018): 131–137.

Chapter 13

1. Wayne L. Westcott, "Resistance Training Is Medicine: Effects of Strength Training on Health," *Current Sports Medicine Reports* 11, no. 4 (2012): 209–216.

2. Brett R. Gordon, Cillian P. McDowell, Mats Hallgren, Jacob D. Meyer, Mark Lyons, and Matthew P. Herring, "Association of Efficacy of Resistance Exercise Training with Depressive Symptoms: Meta-analysis and Meta-regression Analysis of Randomized Clinical Trials," *JAMA Psychiatry* 75, no. 6 (2018): 566–576.

Chapter 14

1. Brad J. Schoenfeld, Mark D. Peterson, Dan Ogborn, Bret Contreras, and Gul T. Sonmez, "Effects of Low- vs. High-Load Resistance Training on Muscle Strength and Hypertrophy in Well-Trained Men," *Journal of Strength and Conditioning Research* 29, no. 10 (2015): 2954–2963.

2. Mike Rosa, email interview by the author, August 18, 2021.

3. Menno Henselmans, "New Science on the Optimal Training Volume: Extreme Training for Extreme Gains?" *Menno Henselmans* (blog), accessed November 14, 2021, https://mennohenselmans.com/optimal-training-volume/.

4. Brad J. Schoenfeld, Daniel Ogborn, and James W. Krieger, "Effects of Resistance Training Frequency on Measures of Muscle Hypertrophy: A Systematic Review and Meta-analysis," *Sports Medicine* 46, no. 11 (November 2016): 1689–1697.

5. Brad Jon Schoenfeld, Jozo Grgic, and James Krieger, "How Many Times per Week Should a Muscle Be Trained to Maximize Muscle Hypertrophy? A Systematic Review and Meta-analysis of Studies Examining the Effects of Resistance Training Frequency," *Journal of Sports Sciences* 37, no. 11 (June 2019): 1286–1295.

6. Florian Egger, Tim Meyer, and Anne Hecksteden, "Interindividual Variation in the Relationship of Different Intensity Markers—a Challenge for Targeted Training Prescriptions," *PLoS ONE* 11, no. 10 (2016), https://doi.org/10.1371/journal .pone.0165010.

7. Eric R. Helms, John Cronin, Adam Storey, and Michael C. Zourdos, "Application of the Repetitions in Reserve-Based Rating of Perceived Exertion Scale for Resistance Training," *Strength and Conditioning Journal* 38, no. 4 (August 2016): 42–49.

8. Daniel A. Hackett, Nathan A. Johnson, Mark Halaki, and Chin-Moi Chow, "A Novel Scale to Assess Resistance-Exercise Effort," *Journal of Sports Sciences* 30, no. 13 (2012): 1405–1413.

9. Tyron Homes, "Macrocycles, Mesocycles and Microcycles: Understanding the 3 Cycles of Periodization," *Training Peaks*, accessed November 14, 2021, https://www.trainingpeaks.com/blog/macrocycles-mesocycles-and-microcycles -understanding-the-3-cycles-of-periodization/.

10. Jozo Grgic, Pavle Mikulic, Hrvoje Podnar, and Zeljko Pedisic, "Effects of Linear and Daily Undulating Periodized Resistance Training Programs on Measures of Muscle Hypertrophy: A Systematic Review and Meta-analysis," *PeerJ* 5 (2017): e3695.

11. Jeff Nippard, "How Hard Should You Train to Build Muscle?" *YouTube*, October 3, 2020, https://www.youtube.com/watch?v=BjyDaxYpW8o.

12. Nippard, "How Hard Should You Train?"

13. Shane R. Schwanbeck, Stephen M. Cornish, Trevor Barss, and Philip D. Chilibeck, "Effects of Training with Free Weights versus Machines on Muscle Mass, Strength, Free Testosterone, and Free Cortisol Levels," *Journal of Strength and Conditioning Research* 34, no. 7 (July 2020): 1851–1859.

14. Jeffrey B. Kreher and Jennifer B Schwartz, "Overtraining Syndrome: A Practical Guide," *Sports Health* 4, no. 2 (March 2012): 128–138.

15. Menno Henselmans, "The Deload Roundtable with Eric Helms, Mike Israetel and Menno Henselmans," *Menno Henselmans* (blog), accessed November 14, 2021, https:// mennohenselmans.com/deload-roundtable/.

16. Jaime Hinzpeter, Álvaro Zamorano, Diego Cuzmar, Miguel Lopez, and Jair Burboa, "Effect of Active versus Passive Recovery on Performance during Intrameet Swimming Competition," *Sports Health* 6, no. 2 (March 2014): 119–121.

17. Menno Henselmans, "The Natural Muscular Potential of Women," *Menno Henselmans* (blog), accessed November 14, 2021, https://mennohenselmans.com/ natural-muscular-potential-women/.

18. Stephen M. Roth, Fred M. Ivey, Greg F. Martel, Jeff T. Lemmer, Diane E. Hurlbut, Eliot L. Siegel, E. Jeffrey Metter, et al., "Muscle Size Responses to Strength Training in Young and Older Men and Women," *Journal of the American Geriatrics Society* 49, no. 11 (November 2001): 1428–1433.

19. Peter M. Tiidus, "Benefits of Estrogen Replacement for Skeletal Muscle Mass and Function in Post-menopausal Females: Evidence from Human and Animal Studies," *Eurasian Journal of Medicine* 43, no. 2 (2011): 109–114.

20. K. M. Haizlip. B. C. Harrison, and L. A. Leinwand, "Sex-Based Differences in Skeletal Muscle Kinetics and Fiber-Type Composition," *Physiology* (Bethesda, MD) 30, no. 1 (January 2015): 30–39.

21. C. S. Fulco, P. B. Rock, S. R. Muza, E. Lammi, A. Cymerman, G. Butterfield, L. G. Moore, B. Braun, and S. F. Lewis, "Slower Fatigue and Faster Recovery of the Adductor Pollicis Muscle in Women Matched for Strength with Men," *Acta Physiologica Scandinavica* 167, no. 3 (November 1999): 233–239.

22. Paul S. Kim, Jerry L. Mayhew, and D. Fred Peterson, "A Modified YMCA Bench Press Test as a Predictor of 1 Repetition Maximum Bench Press Strength," *Journal of Strength and Conditioning Research* 16, no. 3 (August 2002): 440–445.

23. Menno Henselmans, "9 Reasons Why Women Should Not Train Like Men," *Menno Henselmans* (blog), accessed November 14, 2021, https://mennohenselmans.com/why-women-should-not-train-like-men/.

Chapter 15

1. Matthew A Nystoriak and Aruni Bhatnagar, "Cardiovascular Effects and Benefits of Exercise," *Frontiers in Cardiovascular Medicine* 5 (September 2018): 135.

2. John D. Ratey, *Spark: The Revolutionary New Science of Exercise and the Brain* (New York: Little, Brown, 2008), 10.

3. Robert C. Hickson, "Interference of Strength Development by Simultaneously Training for Strength and Endurance," *European Journal of Applied Physiology and Occupational Physiology* 45, no. 2–3 (1980): 255–263.

4. J. Mikkola, H. Rusko, M. Izquierdo, E. M. Gorostiaga, and K. Häkkinen, "Neuromuscular and Cardiovascular Adaptations during Concurrent Strength and Endurance Training in Untrained Men," *International Journal of Sports Medicine* 33, no. 9 (September 2012): 702–710.

5. T. W. Jones, G. Howatson, M. Russell, D. N. French, "Performance and Endocrine Responses to Differing Ratios of Concurrent Strength and Endurance Training," *Journal of Strength and Conditioning Research* 30, no. 3 (March 2016): 693–702.

6. Rebekah R. Estes, Amy Malinowski, Meredith Piacentini, David Thrush, Eric Salley, Cassidy Losey, and Erik Hayes, "The Effect of High Intensity Interval Run Training on Cross-sectional Area of the Vastus Lateralis in Untrained College Students," *International Journal of Exercise Science* 10, no. 1 (2017): 137–145.

7. Jae Hoon Ryu, Il Young Paik, Jin Hee Woo, Ki Ok Shin, Su Youn Cho, and Hee Tae Roh, "Impact of Different Running Distances on Muscle and Lymphocyte DNA Damage in Amateur Marathon Runners," *Journal of Physical Therapy Science* 28, no. 2 (February 2016): 450–455.

8. J. LaForgia, R. T. Withers, and C. J. Gore, "Effects of Exercise Intensity and Duration on the Excess Post-exercise Oxygen Consumption," *Journal of Sports Sciences* 24, no. 12 (December 2006): 1247–1264.

9. S. E. Keating, N. A. Johnson, G. I. Mielke, and J. S. Coombes, "A Systematic Review and Meta-analysis of Interval Training versus Moderate-Intensity Continuous Training on Body Adiposity," *Obesity Reviews* 18, no. 8 (August 2017): 943–964.

10. This is especially true for women, who we now know take longer to recover from *explosive* movements.

Chapter 16

1. Christopher Barakat, Jeremy Pearson, Guillermo Escalante, Bill Campbell, and Eduardo O. De Souza, "Body Recomposition: Can Trained Individuals Build Muscle and Lose Fat at the Same Time?" *Strength and Conditioning Journal* 42, no. 5 (October 2020): 7–21.

2. Emily Rudow, "How I Strengthened and Developed Noticeable Abs," *Better Humans*, June 29, 2020, https://betterhumans.pub/how-i-strengthened-and-developed-noticeable-abs-c8ff4e92318d.

Chapter 17

1. Marie-Pierre St.-Onge, Andrew McReynolds, Zalak B. Trivedi, Amy L. Roberts, Melissa Sy, and Joy Hirsch, "Sleep Restriction Leads to Increased Activation of Brain Regions Sensitive to Food Stimuli," *American Journal of Clinical Nutrition* 95, no. 4 (April 2012): 818–824.

2. Geetali Pradhan, Susan L. Samson, and Yuxiang Sun, "Ghrelin: Much More Than a Hunger Hormone," *Current Opinion in Clinical Nutrition and Metabolic Care* 16, no. 6 (2013): 619–624.

3. Shahrad Taheri, Ling Lin, Diane Austin, Terry Young, and Emmanuel Mignot, "Short Sleep Duration Is Associated with Reduced Leptin, Elevated Ghrelin, and Increased Body Mass Index," *PLoS Medicine* 1, no. 3 (2004), https://www.ncbi.nlm.nih.gov/pmc/articles/PMC535701.

4. Joseph C. Wu, J. Christian Gillin, Monte S. Buchsbaum, Phillip Chen, David B. Keator, Neetika Khosla Wu, Lynn A. Darnall, James H. Fallon, and William E. Bunney, "Frontal Lobe Metabolic Decreases with Sleep Deprivation Not Totally Reversed by Recovery Sleep," *Neuropsychopharmacology* 31, no. 12 (December 2006): 2783–2792.

5. Karine Spiegel, Esra Tasali, Plaman Penev, and Eve Van Cauter, "Brief Communication: Sleep Curtailment in Healthy Young Men Is Associated with Decreased Leptin Levels, Elevated Ghrelin Levels, and Increased Hunger and Appetite," *Annals of Internal Medicine* 141, no. 11 (2004): 846–850.

6. Julia S. Rihm, Mareike M. Menz, Heidrun Schultz, Luca Bruder, Leonhard Schilbach, Sebastian M. Schmid, and Jan Peters, "Sleep Deprivation Selectively Upregulates an Amygdala-Hypothalamic Circuit Involved in Food Reward," *Journal of Neuroscience* 39, no. 5 (2019): 888–899.

7. St.-Onge et al., "Sleep Restriction Leads to Increased Activation."

8. Séverine Lamon, Aimee Morabito, Emily Arentson-Lantz, Olivia Knowles, Grace Elizabeth Vincent, Dominique Condo, Sarah Elizabeth Alexander, Andrew Garnham, Douglas Paddon-Jones, and Brad Aisbett, "The Effect of Acute Sleep Deprivation on Skeletal Muscle Protein Synthesis and the Hormonal Environment," *Physiological Reports* 9, no. 1 (January 2021), https://www.ncbi.nlm.nih.gov/pmc/articles/PMC7785053.

9. Karine Spiegel, Kristen Knutson, Rachel Leproult, Esra Tasali, and Eve Van Cauter, "Sleep Loss: A Novel Risk Factor for Insulin Resistance and Type 2 Diabetes," *Journal of Applied Physiology* 99, no. 55 (November 2005): 2008–2019.

10. Eric Uni and Kimberly Truong, "Sleep Statistics," Sleep Foundation, November 12, 2021, https://www.sleepfoundation.org/how-sleep-works/sleep-facts-statistics.

11. Jeanne F Duffy and Charles A Czeisler, "Effect of Light on Human Circadian Physiology," *Sleep Medicine Clinics* 4, no. 2 (2009): 165–177.

12. Frances O'Callaghan, Olav Muurlink, and Natasha Reid, "Effects of Caffeine on Sleep Quality and Daytime Functioning," *Risk Management and Healthcare Policy* 11 (December 2018): 263–271.

13. Shannon R. Kenney, Andrew Paves, Elizabeth M. Grimaldi, and Joseph Labrie, "Sleep Quality and Alcohol Risk in College Students: Examining the Moderating Effects of Drinking Motives," *Journal of American College Health* 62, no. 5 (2014): 301–308.

14. Amber W. Kinsey and Michael J. Ormsbee, "The Health Impact of Nighttime Eating: Old and New Perspectives," *Nutrients* 7, no. 4 (April 2015): 2648–2662.

15. Danielle Pacheco and Heather Wright, "The Best Temperature for Sleep," Sleep Foundation, June 24, 2021, https://www.sleepfoundation.org/bedroom-environment/best-temperature-for-sleep.

16. Matthew Walker, *Why We Sleep: The New Science of Sleep and Dreams*, read by Steve West (New York: Penguin Books: 2008), audiobook.

Chapter 18

1. Lauren Leavell, "Reasons to Exercise: Weight Neutral Edition," *Lauren Leavell Fitness*, November 23, 2021, https://www.laurenleavellfitness.com/blog/reasonstoexercise.

2. Michelle L. Segar, *No Sweat: How the Simple Science of Motivation Can Bring You a Lifetime of Fitness* (New York: AMACOM, 2015), 194.

3. James Clear, *Atomic Habits: Tiny Changes, Remarkable Results*, read by James Clear (New York: Avery, 2018), audiobook.

Chapter 19

1. Brad Stulberg, "The Myth of One Percent Better Every Day," *Growth Equation*, accessed November 14, 2021, https://thegrowtheq.com/the-myth-of-one-percent-better-every-day.

2. Steven Pressfield, *The War of Art: Break through the Blocks and Win Your Inner Creative Battles* (New York: Rugged Land, 2002), 5.

3. Michigan Medicine, "Behavioral Activation for Depression," accessed November 14, 2021, https://medicine.umich.edu/sites/default/files/content/downloads/Behavioral -Activation-for-Depression.pdf.

4. John D. Ratey, *Spark: The Revolutionary New Science of Exercise and the Brain* (New York: Little, Brown, 2008), 37–38.

5. Michigan Medicine, "Behavioral Activation for Depression."

6. Mel Robbins, *The 5 Second Rule: Transform Your Life, Work, and Confidence with Everyday Courage* (New York: Savio Republic, 2017).

7. Kristin D. Neff and Marissa C. Knox, "Self-Compassion," in *Encyclopedia of Personality and Individual Differences*, ed. Virgil Zeigler-Hill and Todd K. Shackelford (Cham, Switzerland: Springer International, 2017), https://self-compassion.org/wp-content/uploads/2017/09/Neff.Knox2017.pdf.

8. Kristin Neff, "Self-Compassion: An Alternative Conceptualization of a Healthy Attitude toward Oneself," *Self and Identity* 2, no. 2 (2003): 89–90.

9. Cathy M. R. Magnus, Kent C. Kowalski, and Tara-Leigh F. McHugh, "The Role of Self-Compassion in Women's Self-Determined Motives to Exercise and Exercise-Related Outcomes," *Self and Identity* 9, no. 4 (2010): 363.

10. Brittany N. Semenchuk, Shaelyn M. Strachan, and Michelle Fortier, "Self-Compassion and the Self-Regulation of Exercise: Reactions to Recalled Exercise Setbacks," *Journal of Sports and Exercise Psychology* 40, no. 1 (2018): 31–39.

Chapter 20

1. Committee on Physical Activity and Physical Education in the School Environment, Food and Nutrition Board, and Institute of Medicine, "Physical Activity, Fitness, and Physical Education: Effects on Academic Performance," in *Educating the Student Body: Taking Physical Activity and Physical Education to School*, ed. Harold W. Kohl III and Heather D. Cook (Washington, DC: National Academies Press, 2013), https://www .ncbi.nlm.nih.gov/books/NBK201501.

2. Ron Friedman, "Regular Exercise Is Part of Your Job," *Harvard Business Review*, October 3, 2014, https://hbr.org/2014/10/regular-exercise-is-part-of-your-job.

3. Ryan Holiday, "The Timeless Link between Writing and Running and Why It Makes for Better Work," *Observer*, September 6, 2016, https://observer.com/2016/09/the-timeless-link-between-writing-and-running-and-why-it-makes-for-better-work/.

Chapter 21

1. Michael A. Singer, *The Untethered Soul: The Journey beyond Yourself*, read by Peter Berkrot (Oakland: New Harbinger, 2007), audiobook.

2. Eckhart Tolle, *The Power of Now: A Guide to Spiritual Enlightenment*, read by Eckhart Tolle (Vancouver: Namaste and New World Library, 1997), audiobook.

3. Tara Brach, *Radical Acceptance: Embracing Your Life with the Heart of a Buddha* (New York: Bantam Dell, 2003), 93.

4. Evelyn Tribole and Elyse Resch, *Intuitive Eating: A Revolutionary Program That Works* (New York: St. Martin's, 2012).

5. Joseph B Nelson, "Mindful Eating: The Art of Presence while You Eat," *Diabetes Spectrum* 30, no. 3 (August 2017): 171–174.

6. Jon Kabat-Zinn, *Full Catastrophe Living: Using the Wisdom of Your Body and Mind to Face Stress, Pain, and Illness*, read by Jon Kabat-Zinn (New York: Bantam Dell, 1990), audiobook.

Conclusion

1. Robert Greene, *Mastery* (New York: Viking, 2012), 25.

Resources

1. The training plans presented here were created by Mike Rosa, founder of Anabolic Aliens.

Glossary

Automaticity—the state of being where habits become automatic behaviors.

Base metabolic rate—the number of calories the human body needs to perform basic bodily functions.

Body recomposition—the act of eating at maintenance calories or at a slight deficit with the goal of losing body fat while concomitantly gaining lean muscle mass.

Bulking—the act of purposely eating in a caloric surplus with the primary goal of gaining muscle.

Calorie—a unit of energy or the heat needed to raise the temperature of 1 kilogram of water from 0 to 1 degree Celsius.

Carbohydrates—molecularly, a combination of carbon, hydrogen, and oxygen in a 1:2:1 ratio; digested or transformed into glucose (sugars) to be used as energy by the body.

Cardio—cardiovascular exercise; a form of aerobic exercise that require oxygen and elevates the heart rate.

Compound exercises—exercises that work more than one body part at a time.

Cutting—the act of purposely eating in a caloric deficit with the goal of losing body fat.

Deloading period—the reduction of your training load and intensity or stopping entirely on training for a specific period of time.

Dietary fiber—found in plant-based foods that cannot be digested by the body, but as it passes through our systems, it provides us with a myriad of health-related benefits aside from nutrition; consists of soluble fiber, or able to dissolve in water, and insoluble fiber, or unable to dissolve in water.

Extrinsic motivation—the drive to do something to gain an external reward.

Fat-free mass—also referred to as lean body mass and is calculated by taking the total body mass less the fat mass.

Fat mass—the proportion of fat on the body; most commonly taken as a percentage of overall body mass, referred to as body fat percentage.

Fats—the most calorie dense of the macronutrients; stored in the muscles and provide energy to the body, among other benefits; primary types include saturated, unsaturated, and trans.

Goal—the object of a person's ambition or effort.

Habit loop—a feedback loop or cycle consisting of three components—cue, action, reward—that is instrumental in the formation of a habit.

High-intensity interval training—HIIT; short bursts of intense exercise interspersed with periods of low intensity and rest.

Implementation intention—a principle of habit formation that increases the likelihood that a person will perform the action required in the habit loop by setting specific intentions to do so.

Intermittent fasting—the act of giving the body a short break from eating, from a certain number of hours in a given day to a full day or days.

Intrinsic motivation—the internal drive to do something that stems from a need for self-growth.

Intuitive eating—philosophy developed by nutritionists Elyse Resch and Evelyn Tribole for listening to one's body through interoceptive awareness regarding one's relationship to food and hunger.

Isolation exercises—exercises that work a certain body part or area to focus on a specific muscle or joint.

Ketogenic diet—a diet that is very high in fats, moderate in proteins, and low in carbohydrates.

Law of thermodynamics—a law of physics regarding the preservation of energy when added to a system—the energy is either expended or stored.

Low-intensity steady-state training—LISS; exercising at about 40% to 70% of one's maximum heart rate; examples include walking or jogging at a light pace.

Macronutrients—the nutrients the body needs in larger quantities to provide sustained energy; consist of carbohydrates, fats, and proteins.

Maintenance calories—the exact number of calories to support your daily energy expenditure.

Micronutrients—the vitamins and minerals essential to nutritional health.

Muscle failure—occurs when you physically cannot do another repetition; aids in muscle growth.

Non-exercise activity thermogenesis—the ability to burn calories from normal daily activities.

Nutrition timing—the act of paying attention to the timing of when and what you eat, typically before and during workouts.

One-repetition maximum (1RM)—the maximum amount of weight an individual can lift in a single repetition with proper form.

Progressive overload—doing more training work over time to achieve muscle growth (hypertrophy), such as increasing the weight, doing more reps, more sets, and/or slowing down the tempo.

Proteins—molecularly, they are composed of long-chain amino acids and provide certain benefits to the body including building and repairing muscle tissues, improving the immune system and transporting nutrients to different part of the body; founds in animal and plant-based foods.

Recovery—the act of giving the body adequate rest between training sessions; active recovery includes light, non-strenuous exercises and passive recovery involves sitting, sleeping, or barely performing any physical movements.

Refeed days—incorporating certain days during the cutting phase to bring caloric intake back up to maintenance or to eat in a surplus to give the body a break from calorie restriction.

Reps in reserve—the inverse of reps to failure; the number of reps you are still able to perform after completing a set.

Reps to failure—used in weight lifting to calculates the rate of perceived exertion; the number of reps of a particular movement that can be done before hitting muscle failure in a given set.

Resistance training—also referred to as weight training or strength training; uses resistance to cause muscles to contract helping us build strength, power, and muscle.

Self-determination theory—theory that proposes that humans derive their motivation to take action and grow from harnessing three innate psychological needs: competence, autonomy, and relatedness.

Temptation bundling—a habit formation concept developed by behavioral economist Katherine Milkman; a rewards tactic that increases your likelihood of performing an action by pairing an undesired behavior with a desired one.

Thermic effect of food—the increase in a person's metabolic rate by the consumption, digestion, metabolism, and storage of food.

Training frequency—refers to the number of times you work a muscle in a given week.

Training intensity—refers to how hard you're working in the gym and is an important stress variable in building muscular adaptations.

Training volume—the amount of work done in the gym, usually expressed by the number of sets for a given body part, but it can also include the number of reps per week and load (how much weight is being lifted).

Weight—a person's body mass, or how heavy they are, commonly measured in kilograms or pounds.

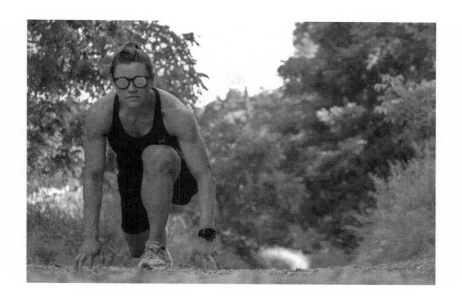

About the Author

EMILY RUDOW is a digital marketer, an entrepreneur, and a fitness writer. She holds a bachelor's degree in business administration from Wilfrid Laurier University. Emily is also an avid long-distance runner. In 2017, she broke a world record by running 74 consecutive half-marathon distances (21.1 kilometers/13.1 miles) while raising over $10,000 for the Canadian Cancer Society.

Since then, she hasn't stopped running. To date, she has run an average of 10 kilometers every day for over four years. She has completed more than 10 marathons (including the Boston Marathon and New York Marathon) and in 2019 came in first in her gender category and third overall in the Haliburton Forest 100 Miler. In 2018, she placed second in her gender category in the Haliburton 50 Miler.

On Emily's blog, *Go Do*, and in *Medium*, she has shared unorthodox training and nutrition tips that have helped thousands of people make transformative changes to their body composition. Emily has built a highly engaged, supportive community and loyal readership on her Instagram, her blog, and *Medium*, receiving emails and messages every day on how her work has affected readers in a positive way. All backed by contemporary academic discourse and the latest psychology, Emily's writings share the most up-to-date scientific literature and research to debunk myths and misinformation being circulated in the fitness industry. In 2017, she launched her #RUN30 challenge, helping hundreds of people develop a consistent running routine.

Emily currently resides in beautiful Vancouver, British Columbia, Canada.